AN ASTROLOGICAL GUIDE TO HEAL YOURSELF

An invitation to reclaim an ancient healing tradition. Learn ways to safeguard health by using natural products available through the bounty of nature.

Blending herbs and astrology together, learn ways to prevent or even heal illnesses.

For healers and astrology buffs alike.

AN ASTROLOGICAL GUIDE TO HEAL YOURSELF

Herbs, Health Foods and Your Zodiac

by

ADA MUIR

With an introductory section on the use of herbs by

JUDE C. WILLIAMS,
MASTER HERBALIST

New Age Books

ISBN: 978-81-7822-230-1

First Indian Edition: Delhi, 2007
Reprinted from: *Healing Herbs & Health Foods of the Zodiac* by
arrangement with Llewellyn Publications, St. Paul, MN 55107, USA
www.llewellyn.com

Published by
NEW AGE BOOKS
A-44 Naraina Phase-I
New Delhi-110 028 (INDIA)
Email: nab@vsnl.in
Website: www.newagebooksindia.com

For Sale in Indian Subcontinent Only

Printed in India
at Shri Jainendra Press
A-45 Naraina Phase-I, New Delhi-110 028

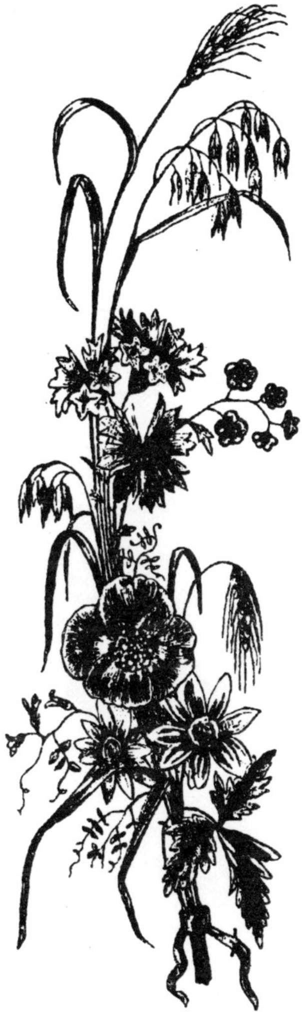

Table of Contents

Section One: Introduction to the Use of Herbs

The Use of Herbs 3
Harvesting the Herbs 13
Basic Remedy Preparation 31

Section Two: The Healing Herbs of the Zodiac

Introduction 51
The Herbs of Aries 53
The Herbs of Taurus 59
The Herbs of Gemini 63
The Herbs of Cancer 67
The Herbs of Leo 71
The Herbs of Virgo 75
The Herbs of Libra 79
The Herbs of Scorpio 83
The Herbs of Sagittarius 87
The Herbs of Capricorn 91
The Herbs of Aquarius 95
The Herbs of Pisces 101

SECTION THREE: HEALTH AND THE SUN SIGNS

Introduction 107
Medical Astrology 109
Health and the Sun Sign 115
The Cell Salts of Aries 119
The Cell Salts of Taurus 123
The Cell Salts of Gemini 127
The Cell Salts of Cancer 131
The Cell Salts of Leo 135
The Cell Salts of Virgo 139
The Cell Salts of Libra 143
The Cell Salts of Scorpio 147
The Cell Salts of Sagittarius 151
The Cell Salts of Capricorn 155
The Cell Salts of Aquarius 159
The Cell Salts of Pisces 163
How to Use Herbs 167
Herbs and Diseases of Common Signs 169
Herbs and Diseases of Fixed Signs 171
Herbs and Diseases of Cardinal Signs 175

Foreword

Healing Herbs and Health Foods of the Zodiac unites two of Earth's oldest traditions, herb lore and astrology, in their modern incarnation.

The Plant Kingdom is the foundation for all life, from it we derive our sustenance and find—as herbalist of old maintained—a cure for every ill. Herbal preparations are the oldest medicines in any culture, and remain the source for most modern drugs. From the rain forests of Brazil to the mossy rocks of the Arctic, Nature provides a wealth of diverse botanicals.

Astrology is our oldest system for understanding and organizing our personal and social world. So a rich heritage of astrological factors in human health has been developed. Physicians of old looked to their patient's horoscopes for guidance to diagnosis and cure disease and directions for health maintenance.

Only recently in human history did we blindly turn away from traditional knowledge, losing our awareness of the astrological factors in disease and the healing powers of herbs. People thought of herbs only as condiments, neglecting not only their medicinal value, but ignoring entirely their ability to act as catalysts to enhance the nutritional value of the foods with which they are blended.

Fortunately, the last twenty years or so have brought about a renaissance. "Alternative" medicine (natural and holistic approaches to healing and health maintenance) and the organic approach to food with a broadened understanding of nutrition have worked together to restore herbs to a place of honor in the kitchen and the medicine cabinet.

As Jude Williams indicates in the first section, herbs are not only readily available in the market place, but you can easily grow a wide variety in your garden or even indoors. Herb lore is rich and fascinating—here you find the gourmet side of living, and discover sources of romance and magical enhancement for every day or special day living. The crafts of growing and compounding herbs are personally enjoyable, and encourage a shift in consciousness that brings the herbalist an inner awareness of the more subtle properties of these magical plants—an awareness that helps bring the herbalist into an active and more spiritual role in diagnosing and healing.

Some readers will note that the astrology in this book is "traditional" rather than "modern." Medicinal astrology relies on traditional planetary relationships and herb correspondences because these ancient relationships are well established and understood.

Ada Muir's contribution to our healing renaissance was to remind us of the important relationship between astrology and herbalism and to give this relationship a contemporary expression. Over 100,000 copies of her *Healing Herbs of the Zodiac* have been sold, making it a minor publishing classic. Combining it with her *Health and the Sun Signs*, and augmenting both with additional information by Master Herbalist Jude Williams, we feel that the Alternative Health spectrum is vastly enhanced.

Health is a personal responsibility, and the fulfillment of that responsibility includes regular consultation with health professionals. However, many healing decisions are made in the kitchen and the herb garden, and it is to that awareness that this book is dedicated.

By Carl Llewellyn Weschcke

SECTION ONE:

INTRODUCTION TO THE USE OF HERBS

BY JUDE C. WILLIAMS

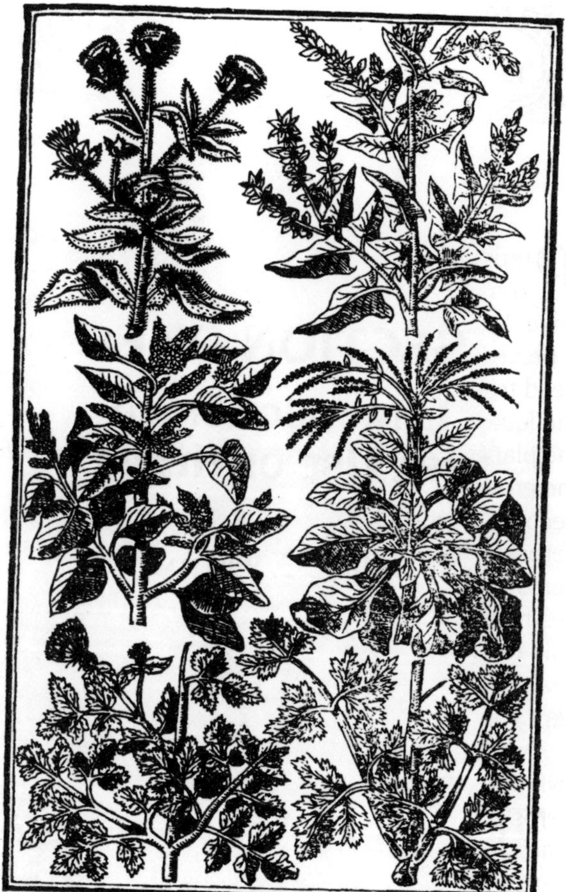

The Use of Herbs

Preparation of herbs for personal use is something that takes some advance knowledge. If you are interested in using the herbs as a preventative measure or as a treatment, you need to know how to identify the plants. One of the fastest ways I know to become familiar with the plants is to grow them. You are then aware of the growing habits and have the time needed to become familiar with the uses of the different herbs. Many times, those who have an interest in herbs but don't have the available space or the desire to grow them become quite knowledgeable by purchasing dried herbs from their local health food store. Just be cautious trying any herb you are not knowledgeable about.

One of the reasons I encourage growing your own herbs is to insure the purity of the product. Herbs purchased from out of the area are sometimes fumigated and all that come from out of the country are definitely fumigated. Most of the vegetables and fruits that you purchase from your local grocery store have been irradiated and sometimes fumigated. So I do encourage anyone interested in protecting their own and their family's health to start gardening and preserving their own food supply. Your diet is the most important way to start safeguarding your health and practicing a preventative health lifestyle.

The use of fruits and vegetables as a health treatment began long ago. So long ago, in fact, that the records are lost in the mists of time. All the oldest herbal books that I have been privileged to read have always had recipes for preparing different food dishes as a treatment for specific illnesses. The importance of the cell salts that are in fruits and vegetables has long been underrated. Our bodies are made up of different minerals and any deficiency causes the body to react in a certain way even unto death. Most of mankind's illnesses are caused by an insufficiency of certain salts and minerals.

The earth has been depleted of most of the minerals needed to grow healthy foods, so we must become aware of how we feed our soils in our gardens to have the vitamins and minerals needed in our foods. This goes back to having a reverence for Mother Earth. We become more balanced in our life as we work to better the little piece of earth that we occupy. We learn the basic way to garden that helps us set new priorities and, surprisingly, is easier. We start by recycling material for our compost and end up becoming more responsible for what we purchase and even how we use things. We become aware of how important all the insects and animals are to the food chain.

The Shakers are responsible for helping the physicians and the public to save and use the herbs in a medicinal manner here in the United States. There are many herb gardens in the process of being recreated now that show how intensively the Shakers did grow herbs for sale. They started out healing by laying on of hands and this was very successful, but they realized that not everyone had the gift of healing in this manner. There were others that needed the healing power of plants. The Shakers were saving vegetable seeds for resale and herb gardening just gradually came into being as they started using the plants for healing members of their communities. They soon became quite successful in selling herb seeds and dried herbs to the public and to pharmaceutical companies.

As folk medicine became popular, there were several other unorthodox schools of medicine that were just as popular. Hydrotherapy was one school. Hydrotherapy, or water cure, became quite popular as they treated diseases using certain mineral springs. This lead many to understand that the minerals could also be used from plants. They understood and made sure that their gardens had the capacity to heal by using natural ways to ensure that the soil in the gardens was healthy. Composting and mulching was already being practiced by the Shakers and they became more proficient in their gardening methods. They started giving booklets with their seeds that explained how to garden.

The American Reformed System started by a Dr. Wooster Beech was one that started substituting the vegetable remedies for chemical treatments. As people became more knowledgeable about gardening and saving seeds for their own use, the business of raising and selling herbs and vegetable seeds to the public became unprofitable for the Shakers. The organization stopped the business on a large scale in 1829. They continued to use herbs for their own remedies.

The history of the Shakers is very interesting and shows how important herbs were for healing in the early 1800's. There are many different gardens that have been recreated that make for a wonderful visit to learn more about the history of the herbs. There are the gardens of Shakertown at Pleasant Hill, Inc. in Harrodsburg, Kentucky; Mount Lebanon Shaker Village in Mount Lebanon, New York; Hancock Shaker Village, Inc. in Pittsfield, Massachusetts; and the gardens at Lower Shaker Village in Enfield, New Hampshire.

The use of vegetables as a health aid does not mean that the use of vegetables heals. The fact that you are building a strong immune system by having a healthy diet causes the healing. Your body heals itself. We are simply being aware that we must keep the immune system healthy and strong enough to fight off the diseases that we are exposed to on a daily basis. So we learn not to underestimate the uses of fruits and vegetables in our diet.

Medicinal herbs use became popular when we realized that not all illnesses can be prevented and we needed help in addition to our ordinary diet. The ancient healers turned to what was on hand and natural. Every tree, flower, shrub, and plant was utilized. This use and experimentation by early herbalists was a deadly, serious occupation. Life and death literally was in the hands and knowledge of those early shamans. We should be thankful, many of our modern medicines were developed through experimentation many centuries ago. We now have many miracle drugs that came directly from early trial and error.

Learning to use herbs in a responsible and helpful way can become a rewarding enterprise. You will find that the more you know, the more you need to know. There are no mysteries to using natural methods. Once you learn the doctrine signatures of the herbs, understanding the use of herbs becomes much easier. Using herbs then becomes a natural part of your life. This knowledge will never be lost and the ability to aid your body in healing will always be there if needed. Learning to treat or prevent illness in your family is very rewarding. When we do something for ourselves, we acquire the self-esteem that helps us in other areas of our life.

Many will say that herbs in and of themselves cannot heal. I couldn't agree more. Most diseases today can be attributed to stress caused by our hectic lifestyles. When we allow our immune system to become depleted through stress, we open our system up to all kinds of illness. Becoming aware of the natural world through the study of herbs helps us become more aware of the responsibility we have to adapt our lives so we can constructively feed our spiritual needs along with our physical needs. We soon realize that we can have the best food, diets, and medical care available and still suffer on a daily basis from one illness or another. We need to fill our spiritual needs.

We become more balanced and stable in our daily life when we learn to take care of the whole person. Body, Spirit, and Mind are integrated and it is essential to treat all three when we become ill. With this knowledge, modern day herbalists have an edge over modern physicians. They have long known that you are treating a whole person and not just the symptoms of a specific disease. This knowledge goes back far into antiquity and is just now starting to get attention from today's medical community.

By becoming aware of the diseases each astrological sun sign has a tendency to develop, we are going one step further in practicing a healthy life style. We learn which illnesses we can prevent by using certain cell salts obtained from herbs and vegetables. The practice of the science of astrology goes far back into the birth of civilization and it makes sense to combine the wisdom of one science with another for our good. So, putting herbs and astrology together is a natural method that can be used to prevent or even heal illness. Even those already familiar with the medicinal use of herbs can benefit by learning about sun signs.

We can make use of the cell salts by being aware of our diets. The herb treatments can be used in many different ways. The most common and easy ways are to learn the basics of preparing herbal tinctures, teas, and salves.

Soon you may not be able to purchase many of the vitamin supplements and herbal products from your drug or health food store. It makes sense to learn all the different ways we can safeguard our health by using the natural products that are available to us through the bounty of Mother Nature. Studies of the properties of herbs soon teach you which herb, vegetable, or fruit contains the vitamins needed for health. You can also learn some of the supplemental ways to get extra needed vitamins.

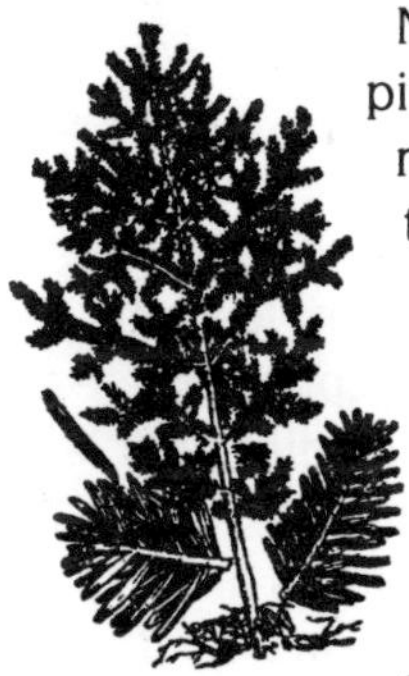

Native Americans used the pine tree as a source of vitamin C. Tea was made from the pine needles. Because the pine has evergreen needles, we need not store a dried source. We can just pick the fresh needles as we need them.

Violets have the largest amount of vitamin A of any known plant, but they aren't available year round. To be able to use herbs during the cold winter months, we need to learn how to dry them for future use. There are many different ways to use so called weeds and wild herbs as well as the more commonly used and grown

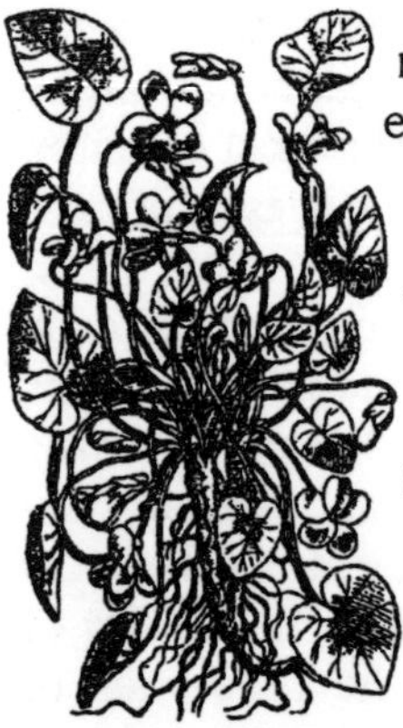

herbs. The use of the culinary herbs allows us to get extra benefits with our meals.

Some wild herbs can supply us with many minerals and vitamins if we just learn to identify and use them. Red clover has a very high mineral and vitamin content—let's learn to use it. Red clover is a member of the pea family and can be used as a pot herb.

Once you become interested in using herbs as supplements, you will have chosen a subject that is never exhausted. You continue to use the plants in many different hobbies or perhaps even as a vocation.

We can learn to use herbs as an income supplement. During slow times in the economy, the knowledge always comes in handy and you are never left unprepared. When you learn to prepare and store your own food supply you are not only saving money, you are providing your family with the highest possible quality of food. The time needed to prepare your fruits and vegetables is minimal compared to the health of someone you love. None of the chemicals are present in the food because you have learned to garden in a natural manner. The foods are also fresher because they are as close as your garden. You may think you are purchasing the highest quality of food from your supermarket, but if you really look at the processes these foods go through you would start growing your own right away.

We live in a world of plenty, yet we have children dying by the thousands from malnutrition. We are supplying them with what we think are good healthy diets. In reality, we are giving them vegetables and fruits with all the enzymes, vitamins, and minerals necessary to our health removed. We need to become responsible in looking at our food source and taking steps to change some of the ways we allow our families to suffer for the convenience of supplying distant markets. We need to love our families enough to put out the extra effort to grow and preserve as much of our own food supply as possible. This is one of the best ways I know to teach future generations that the earth is precious.

Children are sometimes more knowledgeable than adults about the ways we abuse our very life source. They will have to live with our mistakes. Let's learn with them ways to stop the mistreatment of Mother Earth. We can only benefit in the process.

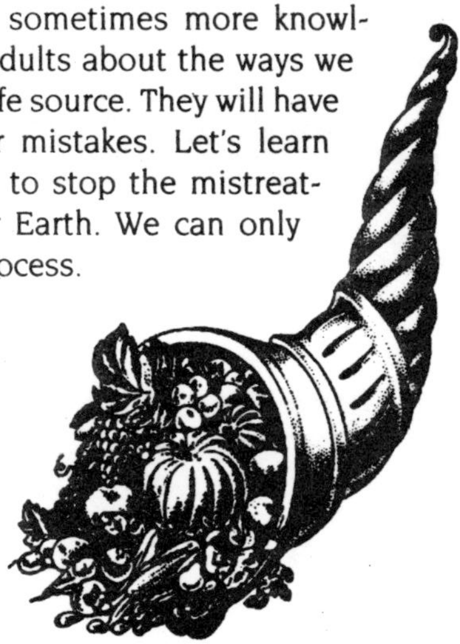

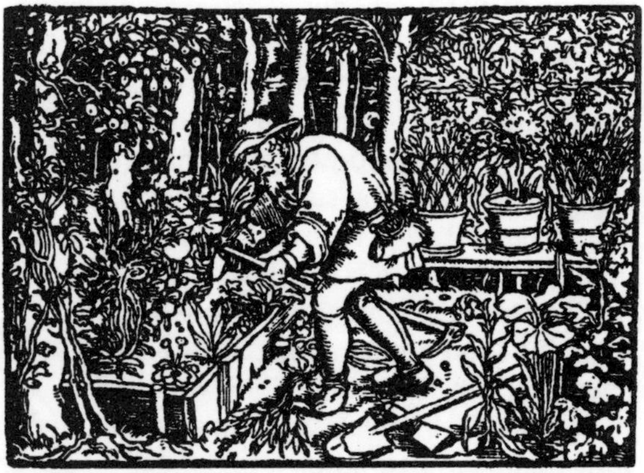

Harvesting the Herbs

Preparing and harvesting the herbs is easy and interesting to do. There are several rules to follow and the basic preparation is the same for most of the herbs. You want to dry the herbs for future use because fresh plants are not available during certain times of the year. Many people prepare and dry herbs for use as tea for pleasure. Medicinal herbs may not always be necessary, but they are useful to have on hand. Generally dried leaves and flowers may be kept for one year. Dried roots can be kept for three to four years. The amount of herbs you need to dry always depends on how often you will use the plant or root. After drying the approximate amount you think you will need the first year, you can dry more or less the following year, depending on use.

Again I want to encourage you to grow your own herbs, even wild herbs. Many herbs are on the endangered species list. We are practicing good husbandry if we purchase herbs from companies that grow them from seed or starts of plants that are not collected from the wild.

By growing herbs, you have the chance to learn the growing habits of the plants and even get acquainted with them in a personal way. Communion with herbs is a common practice. Many shamans and Native Americans still use the reverent way to collect plants. Once they locate the necessary plant, the Medicine Man or Woman will sit next to the plant and meditate after giving a prayer for it. The knowledge then comes to them whether this particular plant is the one needed for the remedy. The use of different herbs is frequently brought to mind and even the source is then known. Before harvesting, the herbs are given a prayer of Thanksgiving.

The strongest plant is never taken and if there is only one of the species growing at a particular spot, the plant is left to propagate and another source is found. Continue the practice of conservation by assisting in the propagation of the plants when using the gifts of Mother Nature. Planting seeds only takes a few minutes and in some measure gives back what we take from the Earth.

Wild herb beds can be very attractive around your home and they sure are useful. If nothing else, you will be able to help novices learn how to identify some of the wild plants that abound in nature. Many schools and parks have a plant identification program in use and this benefits all. The beauty of nature is often unappreciated; growing wild herbs gives you a chance to help others learn to love our natural world.

The best time to harvest leaf herbs is when they are in flower and after there have been several dry days. Always gather herbs after the dew has dried from the plants, but before the sun gets too hot. They hold the most essential oils at that time.

When gathering leaf herbs, you should cut about two thirds of the plant. Gather the stalks and tie in a bundle. Hang the bundles in an area that gets good air circulation until they become brittle. Then remove and crumble the leaves for storage. It is best to use a dark container for storage. Always keep the dried herbs out of direct sunlight. Check the stored herbs in a few days. If moisture has formed, you will need to dry the herbs further. The herbs are useless if mold forms on them. Many times it may be necessary to fast dry the herbs. This can be accomplished by heating them in an oven at a very low temperature. Leave the door open a crack to let the moisture escape. Some herbs, like basil, will turn black if not dried in this manner. Experiment with your herbs and you soon learn the best method. Spread herbs on newspaper or a screen for more effective drying. Don't dry any herbs in the sun. A dry area with good air circulation is the best.

Quite a few recipes call for herb flowers for remedies and these are easy to prepare. Gather the flowers just as they are beginning to open. Place them on a screen to dry. The air circulation is good from top and bottom using a screen. Lay them in a single layer and turn them frequently to ensure that they are thoroughly dry. Then place them in a container that has a tight lid. Make sure you label all containers. You may think that you will remember what you have, but many times the appearance of the dried plants can be misleading. You should also date the container, so that you can replace any herbs that are outdated.

The seeds are the easiest of all to collect. Simply cut the head of the plant after the seeds have ripened and place it in a paper bag. After allowing time for the seeds to dry, simply shake the bag and remove the stems and flower heads. There are many medicinal uses for the seed herbs and the seeds can also be used for a new start the following year.

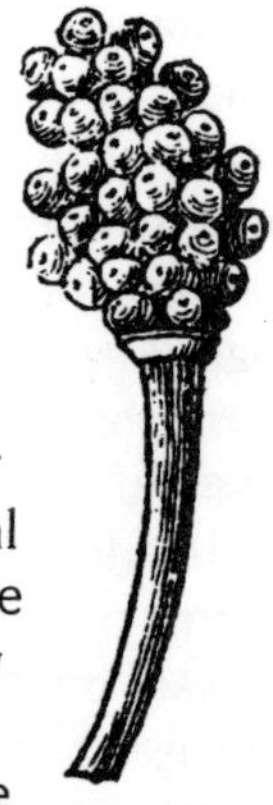

The root herbs take a little more time and effort but are well worth the time spent in gathering and preparing. As a general rule, the roots are dug in the fall. Of course there are a few exceptions, but generally the roots will be collected during the fall months.

After digging the roots, be sure to leave plenty for any future use. Then wash the roots thoroughly using a brush to ensure you get all soil off them. Drain them well and slice the roots lengthwise so that you have thinner strips to dry. Place them in a single layer on a screen. Put the screen in a warm dry area and turn frequently. Low humidity is a must when drying roots.

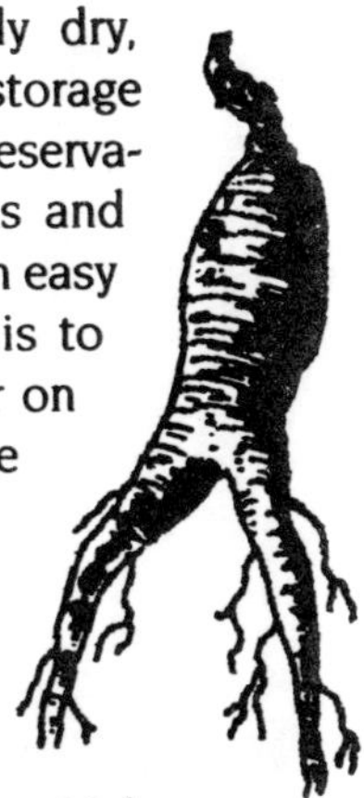

When they are thoroughly dry, place them in an air-tight storage container. You should add a preservative to help protect the roots and bark from insects and mold. An easy way to add the preservative is to put several drops of camphor on an absorbent cloth and place the cloth between waxed paper. Put this in the bottom of the container and place the roots on top. The camphor acts a preservative and keeps bacteria from forming. Make sure you label and date these containers also.

I would only dry enough for your personal use. You can always add to the supply next year. It is better to leave the plant grow than to waste the root if not needed. Because none of the recipes call for a large amount, you would not need to dig large amounts. The one used in our house the most frequently is valerian. I dry a little more of it then I do the other root herbs. I grow enough for our personal use and have no need to gather it wild.

Barks are also easy to dry. Follow the same principle as with the roots. Use the tree branches instead of using bark from the trunk of the tree. Taking bark from the trunk can invite insects and diseases, possibly causing the tree to sicken and die. The inner bark is the part used. Remove the tough outer bark from the limb and the inner bark can then be pulled off in strips. Place the

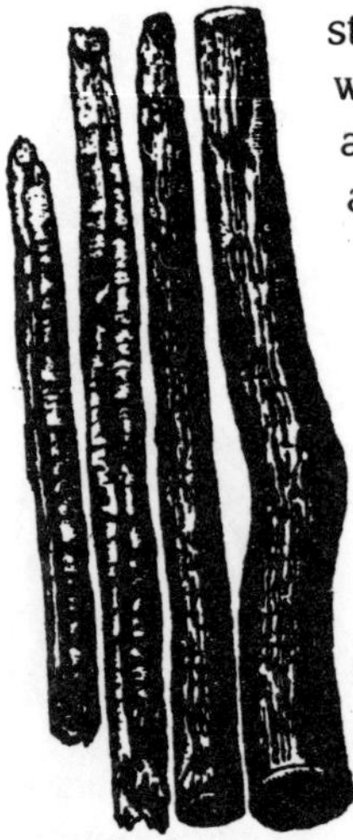

strips on a screen and put in a warm dry area. Low humidity is again necessary and you must add a preservative to ensure no bacteria or mold forms on the bark. Again label and date the storage container.

Balm of Gilead buds are often used for some home remedies and these are gathered in the late winter or very early spring. These are nothing more then buds from the poplar tree (*Populus candicans*) and can be gathered when the buds are covered with the sticky resin. The buds are used in preparing certain salves, cold syrups, and remedies. Dry them on a screen and then store in a air-tight, labeled container.

Herb gathering can go on all year. Spring brings many that are helpful year round. Gather the herbs that are up early in the spring when they are new and tender. Many of the summer herbs need time to ripen and the fall herbs have to reach maturity before they can be gathered. Herbs gathered in very late winter or very early spring are not yet matured.

Once you become proficient in gathering and harvesting herbs, you will find that many of the more common herbs are easy to use and of great value to you and your family.

The following is a partial list of herbs, which includes a brief description of the part of the herb harvested and how it is used.

Anise (*Pimpinella anisum*)
Use the seeds or the leaves. Anise is used primarily as a digestive aid or flavoring for other medicinal teas. The seeds are frequently used for culinary purposes.

Apple (*Pyrus malus*)
Use the whole fruit. It can be dried and used as a tea. It aids in eliminating toxins from the system. If the apple is dried until brittle, it can be placed in the blender and then used as a natural sugar substitute.

Arnica (*Arnica montana*)
The flowers are used to prepare liniments and salves for sore muscles and sprains. It has analgesic properties.

Basil (*Ocimum basilicum*)
The leaves are frequently used as a tonic for the digestive system and as a mild laxative. They are also used to treat headaches and as a mild sedative. The seeds are used in poultices and exhibit an antibacterial effect. There are so many different species of basil that it makes an interesting herb to grow for culinary purposes. Remember we are using all the vegetables and fruits as a preventive measure, including the herbs.

Bee Balm (*Monarda didyma*)
The leaves are are stripped from the stem after drying or picked from the plant before the drying process. Use bee balm for a pleasant tea or for medicinal purposes. It relieves coughs, nausea, sore throat, menstrual cramps, and purifies blood. It is also used to stimulate the liver and spleen. The flavor differs if the plant is harvested before blooming and again after it has bloomed. A drying period of longer then three days may cause the leaves to be discolored. If not dry after three days, hasten the process by drying in an oven at low temperature.

Birch (*Betula ssp.*)
Birch tea relives headaches and many Native Americans used the leaf to prepare a tea for rheumatism. The dried bark was used to treat kidney stones, fevers, and cramps.

Blackberry (*Rubus villosus*)
The leaves, fruit, and root are used. The fruit juice is used to treat diarrhea. The root is frequently used to treat female problems. Gargling with extract made from the leaves remedies sore or swollen throats and it is used to cure sore mouths. Tea made from the leaves is also used to help relieve pain from menstrual cramps.

Boneset (*Eupatorium perfoliatum*)
The leaves and flowers are used to treat colds, coughs, fevers, and flu. This plant grows profusely around our pond and I always enjoy watching it mature. The leaves are the most interesting

part of the plant as they join at the stem and are an attractive dark green.

Borage (*Borago officinalis*)
The leaves and flowers are used. The leaves are used to make a tea for treating depression. The flowers are used to prepare a decoction to relieve fever and to treat bronchitis. It is interesting to note that the herb is listed as officinalis because it is listed by pharmaceutical companies as having a medicinal use.

Burdock (*Arctium lappa*)
The leaves, roots, and seeds are used. The root is a great blood purifier and has been used as such for centuries. The fresh root is often used as a substitution for celery when cooking soups or other dishes. The leaves are gathered in early spring and can be eaten as a raw salad or steamed as a pot herb. They can be used as a poultice for burns, bruises, swelling, and gout. The seeds are added to tea blends as a blood purifier or simply to get the added minerals when using a specific tonic for a treatment. The compounds found in the fresh root do contain certain properties that are shown to inhibit the growth of fungi and bacteria.

Calendula (*Calendula officinalis*)
The flower is harvested. Calendula is used internally as well as externally. It has antibiotic properties and aids in healing wounds. It helps induce sweating and has been used for fevers, flu, and chest ailments.

Celery (*Apium graveolens*)
Tea made from the celery stalk or seed is used to calm nerves and as a sedative.

Chamomile (*Matricaria chamomilla*)
The flower and upper part of the plant are used as a calmative, a sedative, and to relieve headaches and gastrointestinal problems.

Chicory (*Cichorium intybus*)
The flowers are used as a sedative and in skin tonics. The roots are used as a coffee substitute.

Red Clover (*Trifolium pratense*)
The flowers are used for treatment of skin disorders caused by impurities of the blood. The whole plant is used as a pot herb.

Blue Cohosh (*Caulophyllum thalictroides*)
The root is harvested. This herb is considered a woman's herb and is used extensively for problems of the uterus. Persons with high blood pressure should not use this plant because it constricts the blood vessels of the heart.

Coltsfoot (*Tussilago farfara*)
The leaves are used. This herb binds to toxins in the system and removes them. It is used in many remedies for chest complaints and colds and is a good expectorant.

Comfrey (*Symphytum officinale*)
Leaves and roots are used for different remedies. It serves as a demulcent, expectorant, and emollient. The leaves are a great poultice for cuts and

wounds as it has some pain relieving properties and has some antibiotic action.

Corn Silk
Corn silk is one of the strongest herbal diuretics. Tea made from dried corn silk tastes like corn and is used to treat kidney and bladder infections.

Costmary (*Chrysanthemum balsamita*)
The leaves are used. Costmary or Bibleleaf has long been used to repel silverfish and was used as a marker for Bibles to keep insects away. It makes a tea used as a liver tonic.

Dandelion (*Taraxacum officinale*)
The roots, leaves, and flowers are used as a general tonic and for specific treatments.

Elder (*Sambucus canadensis*)
The leaves, fruit, and flowers are used to treat feverish colds and the flu.

Slippery Elm (*Ulmus fulva*)
The inner bark is used in treatments for colds because it is a good expectorant as well as being an emollient. It soothes the bronchial system.

Ephedra (*Ephedra spp.*)
The twigs are used. The powdered form is easy to take as a pill for treatment of asthma and chest complaints. This herb is in many over the counter cold and cough syrups. It is also used in weight reduction. The tea helps break up congestion during severe colds.

Fennel (*Foeniculum vulgare*)
All parts are used. It increases milk production for nursing mothers, is an aid for digestion, and helps calm nervous stomachs.

Gingseng (*Panax quinquefolius*)
The root is used as a tonic for the whole system.

Goldenseal (*Hydrastis canadensis*)
The root is used as tonic for the stomach and liver.

Hollyhock (*Althaea rosea*)
The roots and leaves are used as a substitute for the mallow herb. Use it to treat colds and chest complaints. The leaves can be used as a vegetable dish or in salads.

Horehound (*Marrubium vulgare*)
The flowering top is used as a cough and sore throat treatment. Use it for all bronchial disorders.

Irish Moss (*Chondrus crispus*)
The dried plant is used for colds and chest disorders. It is also used in salves for external treatment of cuts, wounds, and skin disorders.

Lavender (*Lavandula officinalis*)
The leaves and flowers are used to make a sedative tea to treat nervous headaches and tension.

Lemon Balm (*Melissa officinalis*)
The top part of the plant is used. This is a favorite for many people. The tea induces sweating and helps reduce fevers. It is used extensively as a pleasant tasting tea, just for the flavor.

LEMON VERBENA (*Aloysia triphylla*)
The leaves are used to flavor other teas and is used to relax as well as reduce fevers from colds and the flu. Many use it at the first sign of a nervous headache. Helps settle upset tummies.

PRICKLY LETTUCE (*Latuca virosa*)
The gum and leaves are used as a strong sedative. Also, it helps to remove excretions from the bronchial system, making it useful in treating colds and coughs.

LICORICE (*Glycyrrhiza glabra*)
The root is used by women as a treatment during and after change of life. Licorice has estrogen-like properties making it a useful herb for women.

LOBELIA (*Lobelia inflata*)
Harvest the plant after its seed capsules have opened. It is used for bronchial disorders and asthma. Use it with caution as only 50 mg. of the dried herb has caused poisoning symptoms.

MULLEIN (*Verbascum thapsus*)
All parts of the plant are used. This is my favorite herb. It helps in the treatment all bronchial disorders and inhibits certain bacteria. I use it frequently as a treatment for my asthma. Mullein can also be used as a treatment for colds because it has antibiotic properties.

NETTLE (*Urtica dioica*)
The upper part of the plant is used. Strangely enough, tea made from the leaves is used to treat nettle rash. Nettle is also used to treat arthritis pains and as a diuretic.

Pansy (*Viola tricolor*)
The flowers and leaves are used. Pansy is good for treating colds and congestion because it is a mild expectorant. It is great as a heart tonic. Native Americans called this plant heart's ease.

Parsley (*Petroselinum sativum*)
The whole herb is used. This is another common herb that has great value to mankind. Parsley is a wonderful diuretic and is used to treat bladder and kidney infection. Many of the more common herbs can be very useful to us.

Pennyroyal (*Hedeoma pulegioides*)
The leaves are used to treat menstrual cramps because it stimulates the uterine muscles. Pregnant women should not use this under any circumstances. Pennyroyal also relieves upset stomachs and is a mild relaxant.

Peppermint (*Mentha piperita*)
The leaves and flowers are used to treat bronchial disorders. Peppermint is a mild relaxant. In addition, it is good to use for colds and chest complaints because it helps dispel hardened mucus from the system.

Plantain (*Plantago major*)
The leaves are used. It is another common plant that has not been used to full advantage. It makes a good tasting green tea and is used as a diuretic. Plantain has antiseptic properties and is used to remove toxins from the system.

Purslane (*Portulaca oleracea*)
The whole herb above ground is used. Purslane is considered a nuisance plant but nothing could be further from the truth. It is used extensively for the treatment of scours in animals and is a great treatment for kidney problems.

Raspberry (*Rubus idaeus*)
The whole plant is used. This is considered a woman's herb because it is used for female complaints. The leaves and fruit are commonly used for their astringent properties, although the roots can also be used for their antibiotic properties.

Rosemary (*Rosmarinus officinalis*)
Rosemary needles are astringent in nature and are also used to relax the muscles. It is great for relieving tension headaches.

Sage (*Salvia officinalis*)
The top of the plant is used for many different remedies. It's a relaxant, so it is used for nervous headaches and to release tension. The tea is used as a rinse for treatment of dandruff and to prevent graying of hair. Sage also removes catarrh in the bronchial system.

Sheep Sorrel (*Rumex acetosa*)
The leaves are used. This plant has long been used by herbalists to treat cancer and blood ailments. It also cleans the urinary system.

Note: *It is illegal to buy or sell sheep sorrel in Canada. The Canadian and United States FDA have found that sheep sorrel is useful in the treatment of cancer. So bowing to pressure from pharmaceutical companies that stand to make a* *great deal of money from this herb, the Canadian government has decided to remove it from the market because it does have value in treating cancer. I'm sure that the United States will soon follow in removing it from the market.*

SHEPHERD'S PURSE (*Capsella bursa-pastoris*)
The whole plant is used to stop hemorrhages affecting the uterus, stomach, lungs, and kidneys. Shepherd's purse is also used to increase urine flow and helps to remove toxins from the system.

SKULLCAP (*Scutellaria laterifora*)
The above ground parts are used. Skullcap is well known for its sedative properties. Most illnesses are caused by tension; skullcap is added to many remedies for its relaxing properties. Use it to relieve headaches and all nervous disorders.

SOLOMON'S SEAL (*Polygonatum multiflorum*)
The root is used. This herb causes vigorous expectoration during treatment of chest disorders. I had long thought solomon's seal to be poisonous. I have since learned that any plant I had considered poisonous was one I wanted to look at carefully. I have learned that they need to be used with caution but can have a great deal of use for herbalists.

SPEARMINT (*Mentha spicata*)
The leaves and flowering top are used. Spearmint has long been used for treating colic in infants. Adults also use the plant for upsets of the digestive tract. It is also used as a mild diuretic.

STRAWBERRY (*Fragaria vesca*)
Strawberry leaves have long been used as a blood treatment, but there are many uses for strawberry. It has many minerals and is useful for the treatment of scurvy and other mineral deficient blood disorders. Many people use it to treat gout.

SWEET WOODRUFF (*Asperula odorata*)
The part above ground is used. Its odor is not present until you dry the plant. It is used as tonic for the liver and heart and is a good blood purifier.

THYME (*Thymus vulgaris*)
The whole part of the plant above ground is used. It has antiseptic properties and is used for internal as well as external purposes.

VALERIAN (*Valeriana officinalis*)
The root is used to prepare one of the best sedatives to be obtained from herbal sources. It has properties similar to valium—without the side effects. Use with other herbs when treating other illnesses. Illness causes added stress and a sedative is great to add to any treatment. It is also used frequently to treat high blood pressure.

VIOLET (*Viola odorata*)
The flower, leaves, and root are used as a wonderful sedative. The plant has more vitamin A than any known plant, so it is good to use for the vitamin content alone. Violet has long been used as a sedative for older people and particularly for young children. It is also a wonderful tonic.

WILLOW (*Salix spp.*)
Tea made from the leaves, bark, and twigs relieves all kinds of discomfort. It is used extensively as a pain reliever. Willow bark was the first aspirin put out by Bayer and has been used for centuries by Native Americans to relieve pain and discomfort caused by many different illnesses.

WILD YAM (*Dioscorea villosa*)
The root is used extensively by post-menopausal woman because the body treats it like an estrogen. It greatly relieves menopausal symptoms. It is also used as a treatment for asthma and bronchial disorders.

YARROW (*Achillea millefolium*)
The top of the plant is used. Yarrow has some of the same ingredients as aspirin, so the pain reliever is of great help during many illnesses. It also has properties to help blood to clot. It is an astringent and can be used as an external cleanser as well as used internally.

Herbs, as well as vegetables and fruits, can be used to prevent and treat illnesses. It is a subject that you never stop learning about. Used in conjunction with our sun sign, herbs can do nothing but improve our lives by helping us become healthy and whole.

Basic Remedy Preparation

The preparation of salves and tinctures for home use is easy and they are handy to have around the house. Many times, preparing a tincture first and then using it to prepare a salve at a later date is the easiest process. The concept of preparing a tincture is the same whether you are using leaves, flowers, or the root of specific herbs. The only difference is that you would not allow the flowers to stay in the liquid longer than three hours. You are extracting the essence or spirit only of the flower and the time needed is not long.

Flower essences are a well known holistic treatment. There are many different uses and sometimes the use is intuitive. Many practitioners of essence therapy become quite adept at determining what tincture would be best used for a particular patient. Knowledge of the personality and spiritual needs of the person is necessary for the essences to have healing value. Some practitioners are more astute in perceiving those needs than others, but the basic essences are easy to prepare and use.

First, you will learn how to prepare flower essences. With this information, you will better understand the basic preparation of the tinctures.

Preparation of Flower and Herb Essences

Place a small handful of the flower of your choice into a thin glass bowl. Do not use a thicker Pyrex bowl. Cover the flowers with spring water only. Let the bowl sit outdoors in the sun for at least three hours. This allows the healing properties to seep into the water. Strain and fill small sterile bottles half full with the flower water. Fill the remainder of the bottle with brandy. This is a preservative that will keep the remedy for years. Make sure that you label the bottle as to its contents and use. You can mix several different remedies to personalize the treatment.

Herbs can be used in the same manner and can be very helpful to treat many different emotional and spiritual conditions or needs. I will list a few along with the reason for using them.

Aloe Vera (*Aloe vera*)
Use for that burned out feeling.

Angelica (*Angelica archangelica*)
Gives a feeling of protection and helps you to receive guidance from spiritual beings.

Arnica (*Arnica montana*)
Use for treatment of deep shock or disappointment.

Basil (*Ocimum basilicum*)
Helps to polarize and balance sexuality and spirituality.

Blackberry (*Rubus villosus*)
Helps to translate ideas and goals into workable activity.

Borage (*Borago officinalis*)
Builds self-confidence.

Calendula (*Calendula officinalis*)
Helps to put warmth into conversation or social dealing.

Cayenne (*Capsicum frutescens*)
Helps you to accept changes and move toward a definite goal.

Chamomile (*Matricaria chamomilla*)
Gives you a serene disposition.

Red Clover (*Trifolium pratense*)
Imparts calm and steady behavior and helps you to become more self-aware and self-contained.

Black Cohosh (*Cimicifuga racemosa*)
Gives you the courage to confront abusive or threatening situations.

Dandelion (*Taraxacum officinale*)
Gives you plenty of energy and helps to balance inner forces.

Dill (*Anethum graveolens*)
Helps you to appreciate and enjoy all the gifts of life on a daily basis.

Echinacea (*Echinacea angustifolia*)
Heals feelings that have been shattered by trauma.

Evening Primrose (*Oenothera biennis*)
Helps to form committed relationships.

Garlic (*Allium sativum*)
Gives you a sense of wholeness.

Goldenrod (*Solidago spp.*)
Helps balance inner sense of self with social consciousness.

Golden Yarrow (*Achillea clytedata*)
Helps to heal tendency to withdraw from social contact.

Iris (*Iris douglasiana*)
Places you in touch with higher sensitivities and helps you express artistic abilities.

Lavender (*Lavandula officinalis*)
Gives spiritual awareness and sensitivity.

Mallow (*Malva spp.*)
Helps you reach out to others.

Milkweed (*Asclepias syriaca*)
Gives the strength of ego necessary to stop dependency on food, drugs, or alcohol.

Mugwort (*Artemisia vulgaris*)
Allows you to harmonize physic forces.

Mullein (*Verbascum spp.*)
Gives strong sense of conscience and truthfulness.

Nasturtium (*Tropaeolum majus*)
Gives radiant warmth that you are able to impart to others and attracts others to you.

Pennyroyal (*Hedeoma pulegioides*)
Gives you clarity of thought.

Peppermint (*Mentha piperita*)
Stops mental lethargy and helps balance metabolism which can deplete your mental forces.

Pink Yarrow (*Achillea millefolium var. rubra*)
Gives loving awareness of others and stops self absorbency.

Queen Anne's Lace (*Daucus carota*)
Gives spiritual insight and helps integrate physic abilities with spirituality.

Rosemary (*Rosmarinus officinalis*)
Helps correct poor connection of soul and spirit with the physical body and improves memory.

Sage (*Salvia officinalis*)
Gives ability to perceive higher purpose in life.

St. John's Wort (*Hypericum perforatum*)
Illuminates consciousness and gives strength to deal with disturbed dreams and physic experiences.

Scotch Broom (*Cytisus scoparius*)
Makes you feel optimistic about the world and happenings in general.

SELF-HEAL (*Prunella vulgaris*)
Causes healing from within and sense of wholeness.

SUNFLOWER (*Helianthus annuus*)
Gives balanced sense of individuality.

TANSY (*Tanacetum vulgare*)
Helps you to become purposeful in action toward goals.

TRUMPET VINE (*Campsis tagliabuana*)
Gives you freedom to express yourself verbally.

VIOLET (*Viola odorata*)
Elevates spiritual perspective and makes you highly perceptive.

YARROW (*Achillea millefolium*)
Creates beneficial healing forces and helps you to have compassionate awareness of others.

YERBA SANTA (*Eriodictyon californicum*)
Frees up your emotions so you can feel a full range of emotions.

This is just a partial list and you may want to follow it up with further studies. The principle is the same as the Bach Remedies, but using specific herbal flowers and leaves in place of the more common flower remedies. Dosage would be several drops under the tongue when needed.

Preparation of Tinctures

The preparation of the tinctures is about the same except you would be allowing the herb to steep in the base for several weeks in the sun. The base may be an oil or alcohol. Any of the oils found in your home are fine to use. Olive oil is the most common used, but vegetable oil and almond oil are also fine. Just don't use any of the drying oils such as linseed oil.

You are preparing the oil based tincture to use as is or possibly to use in a salve. The oil base is the only tincture that you would use to prepare the salves. The oil based tincture has no preservative, so you will need to add one to keep it free of bacteria. The salves are used to heal the skin and must be completely free of bacteria.

Simply place the herb of choice into a pint jar. The amount used depends on the amount you have available. Pour the oil of choice over the herb, covering it. Place the jar in the sun and allow the mixture to steep for several weeks. Strain out the herb and add preservative to the oil to keep the product pure.

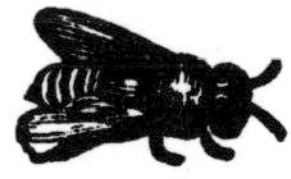

Honey is a great preservative and you only need to add several tablespoons to the oil. Or two vitamin E capsules may be broken open and added as this also is a great preservative. Another possible preservative to use is the tincture of benzoin. Tincture of benzoin can be purchased from your local druggist. Add about a half a teaspoon of benzoin for each pint of oil used. Be sure to label the container as to ingredients, date, and future use. Any herb can be used; there are many books that give instruction on the uses of different herb salves.

Alcohol Based Tinctures

These tinctures are to be used internally. Because you are using alcohol as the base, you will need no other preservatives because alcohol is an excellent preservative. Alcohol based tinctures are also easy to make and use. Simply add the herb of choice to a pint or quart jar. Again the amount of herb would depend on the amount you wish to make and the amount of herb available to you. Pour in enough alcohol to cover the herb. I prefer to use vodka because it has the least noticeable taste. Cover jar and place in the sun. Let mixture steep for several weeks before straining. Label the jar as to contents and dosage.

Many people like to make their tinctures faster and this is easy to do. After filling the jar with the herb and alcohol mixture, place the jar in a pan of water. Bring water to a simmer and allow to simmer until the mixture has reached the desired strength. You will be able to open the jar from time to time and smell to check the mixture's strength. Heating the mixture draws out the medicinal properties of the herb for use. The sun allows the same process and many people like the sun to do all the work.

You would use this tincture to treat headaches, colds, or any simple illness where herbs are used. Use droppers of the tincture as an addition to teas or juice. Many times if the tincture has an unpleasant taste or odor you can fill a gelatin capsule, using an eyedropper, and take with water. Buy the capsules from your local health food store. Dosage depends on the particular herb used and the illness. Generally, several would be sufficient.

Many skin ailments can be treated using an alcohol based tincture. One that comes to mind immediately is valerian. We use this tincture for headaches and as an external application for poison ivy and rashes. It starts drying up the poison ivy immediately and is the only thing that works for my husband's headaches.

Basic Salve Preparation

Herbal salves are great for treating different skin problems. You can prepare the salve as thick as desired and also use it as a lotion for long term, daily use. In preparing the lotions, you make them a little thinner so they are easy to apply. Use beeswax to thicken the tinctures. The dosage would be about two tablespoons of beeswax for each pint of tincture. Test the thickness by placing one tablespoon of the salve into the refrigerator until cool and stiff. If it is too thick, add a little more oil. If it is too thin, add a little more melted beeswax.

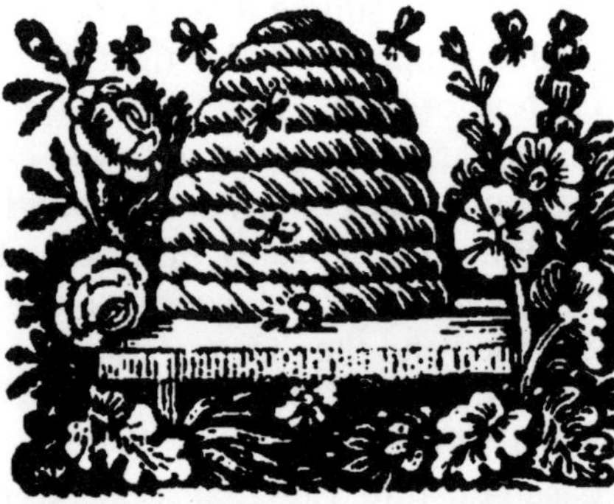

I purchase the beeswax from a local beekeeper in ten pound blocks. Heat and strain the wax, then pour it into pint jars to harden. It keeps for years and I use it by placing an open jar into the microwave long enough to melt the wax needed. I then can just cover the jar and put it away for future use. I don't have to wash any pans and the wax is easy to reuse at a moment's notice.

To prepare the salve from the oil based tincture, just heat the tincture in a stainless steel pan and add enough melted beeswax to reach desired thickness. Because you have already added your preservative to the tincture, there's no need to add more. Test for thickness and store in a sterile large mouth container. Label the container with ingredients and the intended use. These salves keep for years and are easy to store in your medicine cabinet.

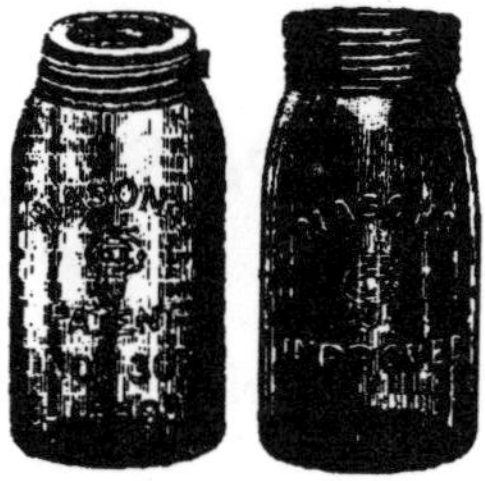

To prepare the salves using fresh herbs, just bring two cups of oil to almost boiling and add a large handful of the herb of choice. Simmer the mixture, depending on the herbs used, for anywhere from 20 minutes to three hours. Then cover the pan and allow herbs to steep until cool. Strain out the herbs and reheat the oil, then add the preservative.

You will need to add a preservative to the fresh herb salve to protect the purity. Add vitamin E capsules, honey, or tincture of benzoin. It is important to add the preservative to keep the mixture from developing bacteria. Finally, add beeswax and stir until the mixture is cool and thickened. Test for consistency and place the salve into a sterile container. Remember to label the container with its contents and use.

Preparing Herb Roots for Salves

The roots of herbs have long been used in salves and these salves are easy to prepare. The roots can be used either dried or fresh. We will assume that you will be using dried herb root. The process is the same as preparing the tincture salves. Chop or slice the root into oil and simmer for at least three hours at a low temperature. Or you can place the root mixture into the oven at a very low temperature to prepare. Leave in the oven anywhere from three to five hours. The heat must be very low to allow time for the healing properties to be drawn from the herb root. A longer extraction time is necessary with the roots than with the leaves or flowers. After slowly and steadily heating the mixture, allow it to steep until cool. Then strain out the roots, reheat the oil, and add your preservative and beeswax. Test the mixture for consistency before placing it in a sterile container. Always label the container as to its contents and use.

Many salves can be made by adding lanolin to the base oil. Lanolin is a healing substance in itself and can be added to any salve for external use. Just add a tablespoon of lanolin to the oil mixture before reheating it.

Use the salves and tinctures for simple skin disorders or injuries that you would be able to treat yourself at home. For more serious injuries, you would need to consult with your physician. The purpose of using these home remedies is to prevent many of the chemicals that are in preparations sold over the counter from being applied to the skin. The skin absorbs everything we put on it and is our first defense against the invasion of chemicals. If these chemicals enter our body, they will be stored in our organs and can possibly cause health problems later on. By using natural products we are taking the first step in defending our health.

Tea Preparation

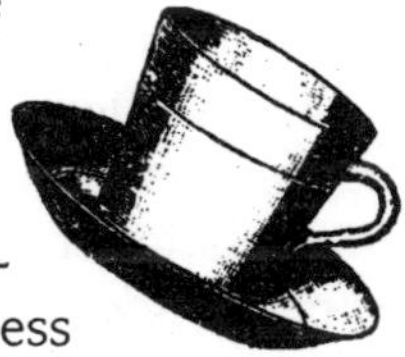

One of the easiest ways to use medicinal herbs is in the form of tea. Preparing herbal tea is easy. First, remember that dried herbs are more concentrated, so you need to use less when preparing tea. Fresh herbs have much more bulk so you would use more when preparing tea. The general rule of thumb is to use one tablespoon of fresh herb or one teaspoon of the dried for each cup of boiling water. You really are better off use less rather than more. So if you are unsure of the dosage, always be on the safe side and use less. We each have different allergies and until you know completely what you are allergic to, use less.

Never boil leaf herbs. This destroys the usefulness of the herbal properties. You need to steep the herb in very hot water for about 10 to 15 minutes, covered, to extract the healing properties from the herbs. You then strain the tea and sweeten to taste. If you are using more then one herb to prepare the tea, you need to premix the herbs and then use one teaspoon of the dried herb mix to one cup of boiling water. It is best to prepare each cup as you need it rather than preparing large amounts of tea that you would have to reheat. Reheating can destroy some of the properties needed.

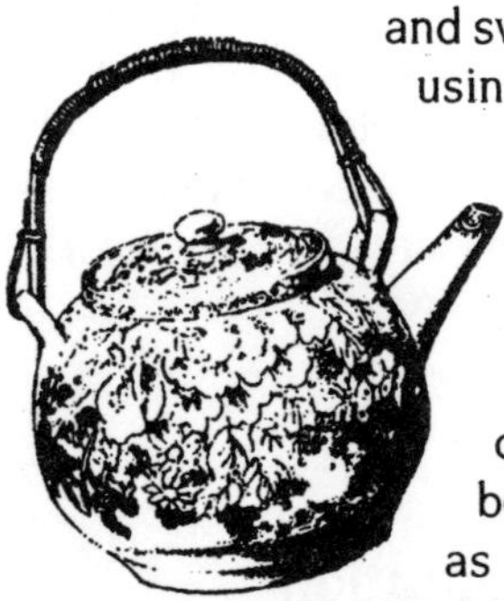

Preparation of teas using the roots is a different process and you need to become proficient in preparing those also. Some basic knowledge is necessary to know why you are using a different method. Any hard substance, such as roots, requires more time to extract the properties of the herbs.

This extraction can be accomplished in several different ways. You can add the roots to water and bring the mixture to a boil, simmer for several hours, and then allow the mixture to sit covered until cool. Keep the liquid covered to ensure that the helpful properties extracted from the herb don't evaporate out. After cooling the mixture thoroughly, strain out the roots, pour the extract into a labeled container, and then refrigerate it.

You may then use this liquid extract by adding about one tablespoon to one cup of hot water as a treatment or tonic. Leaf herbs may be added to this tea and allowed to steep for the 10 to 15 minutes necessary. Again strain and sweeten tea as desired.

Another way to extract the properties needed from the roots is to place the sliced dried root of the herb into the water and place in an oven at a very low temperature. Leave mixture in the oven, covered, for several hours or sometimes overnight. This is a slower process and sometimes, if the mixture is put into the oven late at night, it can be ready for further processing the next morning. I use both methods depending on the time I have available.

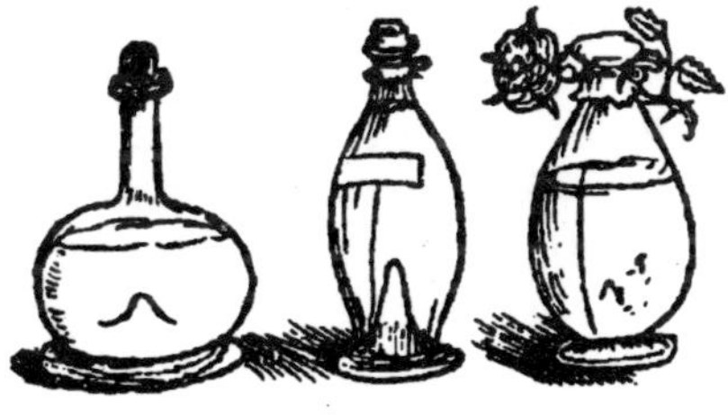

The resulting liquid is easy to store. It is best to add a preservative to the mixture to ensure no bacteria forms. This can be accomplished by adding honey and reheating the mixture, or by adding tincture of benzoin. This would not be necessary if the amount of extract is small and you will be using the liquid within the next few days. Many times, the amount will be used for several months and you would need to add the preservative. You may want to extract the properties using vinegar. This is accomplished the same way as using the water.

Preparing cough syrups sometimes requires you to use some of the root herbs. Prepare the root herbs in the same manner as for tea, adding any of the leaf herbs in the last hour of extraction. The mixture is then strained and an equal amount of honey is added and reheated for another 30 minutes at a very low heat. Additional flavoring may be needed as some of the mixtures can be distasteful. I use wild cherry flavoring for mine. The mixture will thicken as it cools. Refrigerate and use as needed for coughs and colds.

The mixture can also be used as a base for cough drops. Use your favorite hard candy recipe, substituting herbal extract for the liquid called for in the recipe. Wrap the hard drops in cellophane or roll in powdered sugar to keep them from sticking to each other and you have your cough drops. These can also be eaten as candy. If you are using leaf herbs, you need to steep the herb in the boiling water until cool, then proceed with preparing the hard candy. You may use honey or sugar according to the recipe. The following is an easy recipe you may want to try.

Combine the following ingredients:

¾ cup of herbal tea or root extract
2 cups sugar
⅔ cup light corn syrup

Bring mixture to a boil, cover, and allow to boil for two minutes. Using a candy thermometer, measure the temperature of the mixture. When the liquid reaches 285°, remove it from the heat and allow it to sit without stirring until temperature drops to 260°. Add food coloring and citric acid at this time if desired.

Note: Temperatures above 260° will destroy the citric acid. Pour into molds and allow to harden. Store cough drops.

One of the pleasures of preparing and using herbs is the experimentation involved. You soon learn which herbs are the most valuable by learning to prepare them in different ways. Practice always makes perfect, so the more often you use different methods to prepare the herbs, the more you learn. You quickly become used to preparing and using herbs and you may even be surprised to find yourself using herbs in many different ways on a daily basis.

There are many ways to use herbs on a daily basis for preventive health care. Mouth wash, toothpaste, soap, shampoo, and hand lotion are just a few items that are safer and more economical to use if you learn to prepare them yourself. Your whole family benefits and you are helping them to appreciate some of nature's gifts.

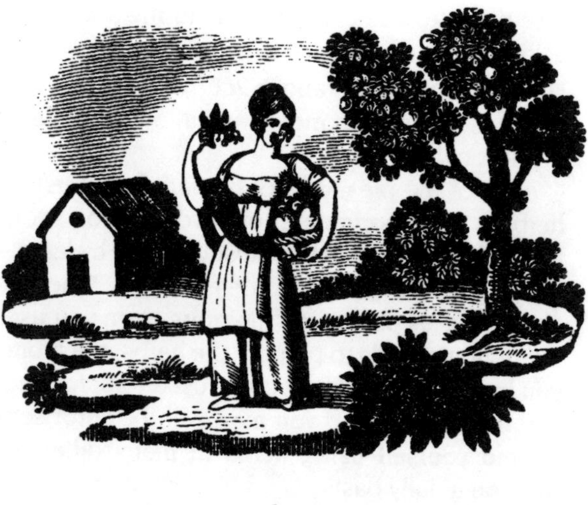

SECTION TWO:
THE HEALING HERBS OF THE ZODIAC

BY ADA MUIR

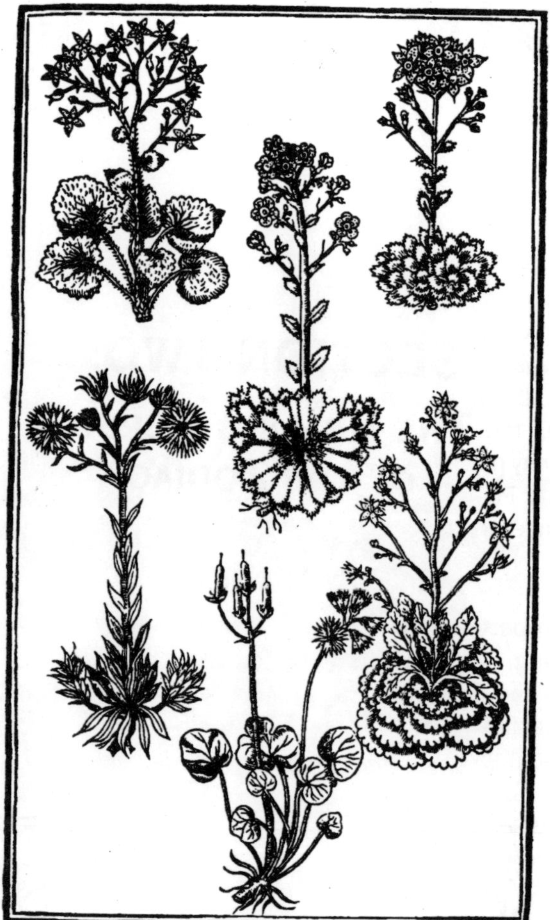

Introduction

Dating from Hippocrates, who wrote in 460 BC and who is recognized as the founder of the art of healing, the properties and values of every wayside herb, tree, and shrub have been known.

It was formerly the duty of every person studying the art of medicine to be able to recognize every plant, understand its virtues, its Zodiacal sign and Planetary ruler, and see that it was gathered under the most favorable planetary conditions.

Nowadays the herbalist knows nothing of this, except in a few cases, but must study the properties of herbs from textbooks and apply them according to the symptoms of disease seen in the patient; and in this way is in danger of making as many mistakes in diagnosis and treatment as the medical doctor.

To give one instance, a friend was made very sick after taking a herbal compound containing barberry, an Aries herb. This had been very successful in the treatment of others suffering similarly, but the cause of the failure in her case was that Jupiter was her afflicting planet and she needed only those herbs in harmony with

Jupiter. Consequently, giving her a Martial herb only intensified the complaint, just as adverse aspects between Mars and Jupiter in a birth chart indicate intensity.

Then herbalists, in their compounding of herbs, often combine them irrespective of planetary laws and the active principal of one will counteract the active principal of another, which, if not injurious, is to say the least, wasteful.

The underlying cause of every disease is indicated in the birth chart as well as the weakness and strength of every organ of the body; for each of the twelve houses of the birth chart governs a definite part of the body.

The study of the Zodiacal rulership of plant life is an introduction to the study of medical astrology and as such should be of great assistance to students of that branch of the science.

The Herbs of Aries

The first house of the horoscope is ruled by Aries and since this describes the head and face in Natal astrology, it follows that the complaints of Aries are primarily complaints of the head and face.

The Sun enters Aries on March 20 and leaves it on April 20 each year. Mars is the planetary ruler of Aries, so those born while the Sun is in Aries, especially if born in the morning, display the martial characteristics of desiring to rule and lead.

The complaints of Aries are of an inflammatory or feverish type, the most common being headache, toothache, neuralgia, gum-boils, ringworm, smallpox (not the modern form of this disease, which is best designated as pimple-pox), mumps, polypus, and burns or scars on the head and face.

The herbs of Mars, (the planetary ruler), being fiery, will help in some cases on the principle that fire will drive out fire by consuming everything inflammable.

It is also true that a fire may be extinguished rather than burned out and so, in some instances, it is better to use the soothing Venus herbs or the cooling and contracting Saturnine herbs, of which more will be said later.

Of the herbs of Aries, the best known are:

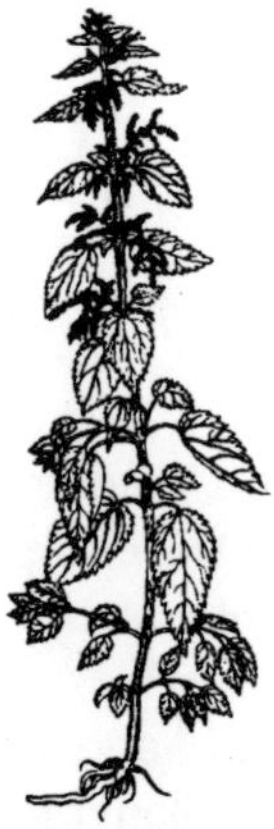

NETTLES

NETTLES will check the flow of blood, is useful as a gargle for a sore mouth, and will stop the nose bleeding, either by snuffing the dried powdered herb up the nostrils, or using as a tea. It is a good spring tonic and blood purifier.

BROOM TEA is a headache cure and the green juice will cure toothaches. If made into an ointment and rubbed well into the scalp, it aids hair growth. It should not be used if Mars and Jupiter are afflicted.

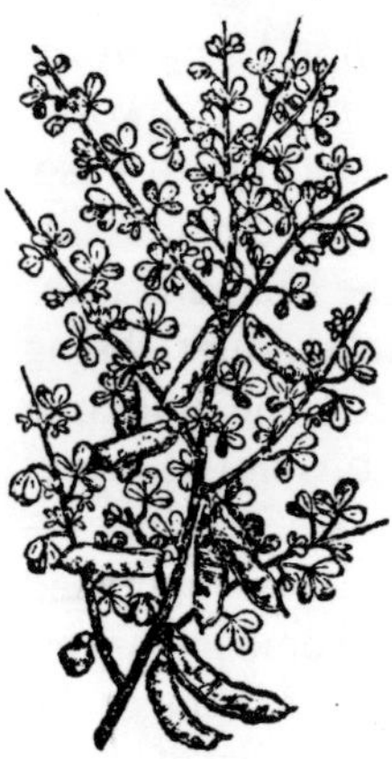

BROOM

GENTIAN is well known as an appetizer and tonic, but it may also be used in the same way as hops. As a tea, it is a blood purifier; wounds bathed with it are cleansed and healed.

Cayenne is an excellent cure for nosebleeding, taken as a tea. Mixed with sage, it is a remedy for nervous headache.

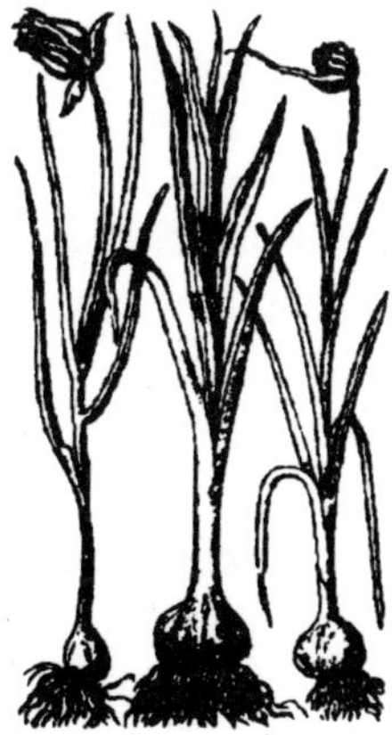

Garlic

Garlic is valuable for treating pains in the ears. For this purpose the expressed juice is placed in the ears. As a poultice, garlic is excellent for the treatment of swellings.

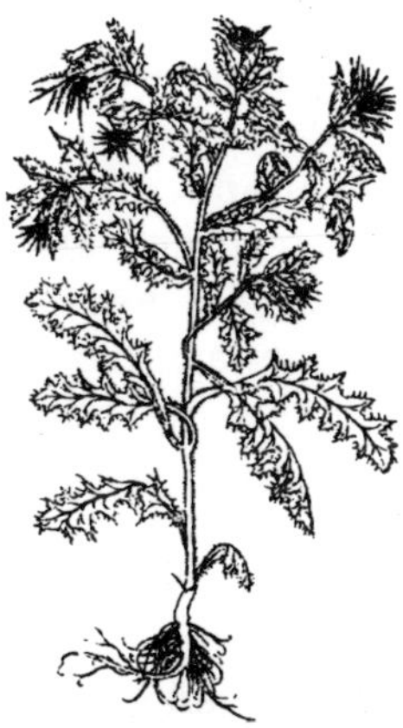

Blessed Thistle

Blessed Thistle is one of the best Aries and Mars plants. Used as a tea, it will relieve giddiness and swimming pains in the head, clear the blood, improve the complexion, and relieve ringworm and itch. It strengthens the memory, and is valuable as a relief for deafness.

Honeysuckle, made into an ointment, is good for massaging the back of the neck in cases of nervous headache, neuralgia, and itch.

Hops are especially good for sleeplessness, used either in a pillow stuffed with the bloom and sleeping upon it, or as a tea, which should be drunk at bedtime. As a wash for ringworm and scabs on the head, it has no equal. It can also be made into an ointment and used for similar complaints.

For Astrological Students

While each Zodiac Sign gives a general idea of the disease, the interplanetary vibrations give a more particular indication. For instance, in Aries subjects, if Mars is afflicted with Mercury, headaches and neuralgic pains are experienced and a nervine such as hops will give relief.

Mars and Venus afflicted incline towards bad habits and scrofulous disease and, for those, cleansing and antiseptic Venus herbs, or the cooling herbs of Saturn, are best.

Mars and Jupiter indicate a disordered liver and here the Jupiter herbs, or those under the rulership of Sagittarius or Pisces must be used.

Mars and the Sun induce fever and either Martial or Venus herbs are useful here.

Mars and Saturn give rheumatic afflictions and the herbs of Mars will stimulate.

Mars and Neptune give disturbances of the astral fluids, as well as scrofulous complaints, and here Mars and Venus herbs combined will give relief.

Ill health is an indication of self limitations.

The signs of the Zodiac give the history of these limitations as they tell of personal bias, fluctuating emotions, unruly desires and wandering thoughts.

The healing herbs of the Zodiac will modify physical conditions, but if the inner cause of the physical condition is understood and character strengthened at the same time, relief will be permanent.

The desires of The Past are responsible for present planetary aspects in our birth charts, as well as for our physical limitations.

The Desires of The Present are ever making our future horoscopes. We can purify these if we will, for we are each a ray from the Heart of all things, and always free to choose our thoughts—the makers of our destiny.

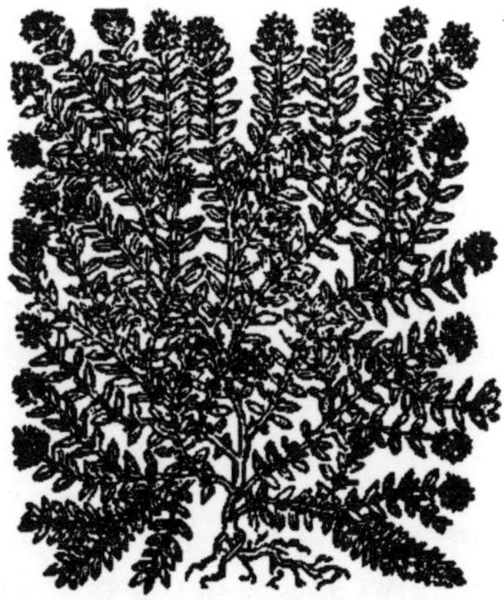

THYME

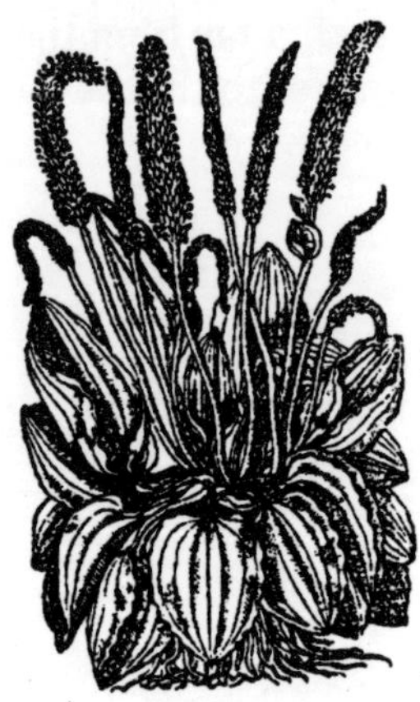

PLANTAIN

The Herbs of Taurus

The second house of the Zodiac, the house of possessions, is ruled by Taurus, and this sign rules the neck and throat, so that the complaints of Taurus are primarily complaints of the neck and throat.

The Sun enters Taurus on April 20 and leaves about May 20. Venus is the planetary ruler. Those born in the morning during that period display the Venusian characteristics of desiring to possess and protect their possessions.

The complaints of Taurus are due to excesses, often of an emotional nature, but sometimes over-indulgence in eating and drinking. The most common are scrofula or King's evil, wens, sore throat, quinsy, abscesses, enlarged tonsils, ague, goiter and bronchial afflictions.

The herbs of Venus purify the blood and keep the sweat glands open, thus allowing the poisonous ferments which have been generated in the body through excesses, emotional or otherwise, to leave the body through the skin.

THE BEST KNOWN HERBS OF TAURUS ARE:

THYME is good for hysteria and is said to inspire courage. It is best used for flavoring for soups or salads.

Plantain made into an ointment is a remedy for scrofula or King's evil.

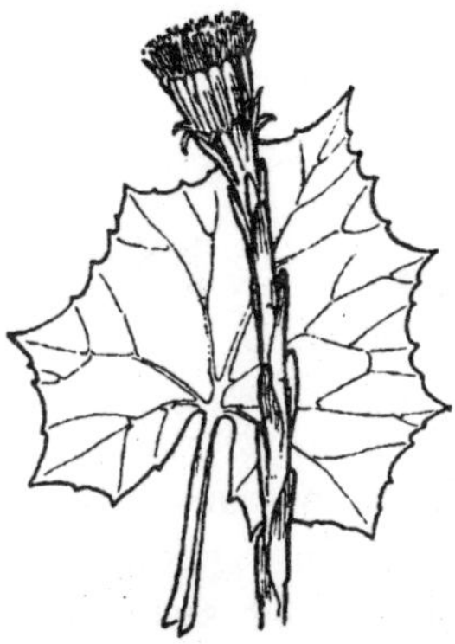

Coltsfoot

Coltsfoot is good for hoarseness, coughs and colds. Use one ounce to one pint of water, sweetened with honey. It will relieve scrofula if taken freely.

Bearberry (Uva Ursi), has no equal for chronic throat affections. The bark should be soaked in water and, as it draws the strength out, should be poured off and drunk; fresh water being then added until the bark gives off no further strength.

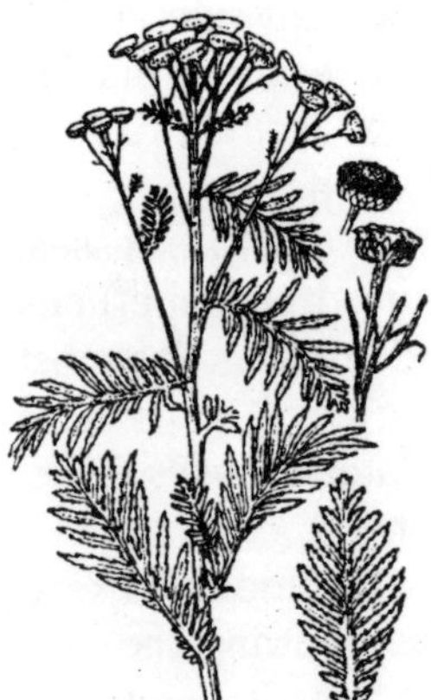

Tansy

Tansy will break up a cold if taken at bedtime, as it causes perspiration. The flowers, dried powdered and mixed with honey, will destroy worms. It is good for those suffering from periodical throat affections.

Sage is the best known and probably the most valuable of the Taurus herbs. A tea made from it will allay emotional excitement and dizziness. Mixed with vinegar, it is a gargle for sore throats, and is one of the best remedies for the mother who wishes to wean her baby, as it prevents food being converted into milk. It strengthens the nervous system and is said to lengthen life. Dose: A teaspoonful in a half-pint of water. Steep for 24 hours but do not boil. Drink a teacup full at night and in the morning.

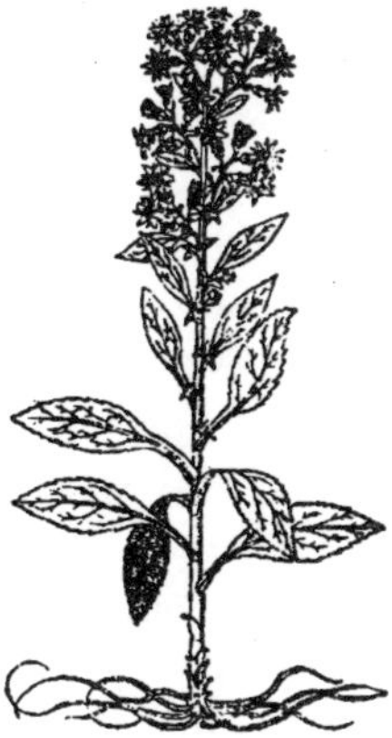

GOLDENROD

GOLDENROD, applied externally, either as an ointment or poultice, will heal ulcers and, as a drink, will heal ulcers in the mouth and throat. It is an excellent tonic for the gums, used strong as a wash or weaker as a drink.

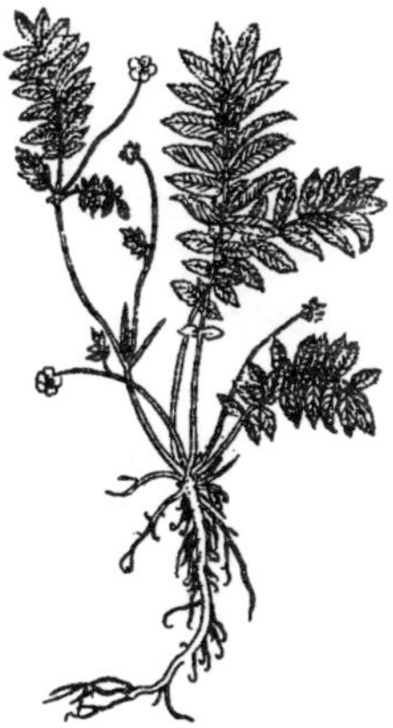

SILVERWEED

SILVERWEED, sweetened with honey, is an excellent gargle for weak and sore throats. Used as a tea it will relieve ague, as it drives the excess water out of the blood.

For Astrological Students

While the zodiacal signs give a general idea of the disease, the interplanetary vibrations give a more specialized indication. For instance, in Taurus subject, if Venus is afflicted with Mars, scrofulous complaints through bad habits or contamination with others so afflicted will be the result. Outward and inward applications of Taurus herbs will be necessary to effect a cure.

Venus afflicted with Mercury by progression will result in neurasthenia and a combination of Taurus and Gemini herbs will give relief, or Taurus herbs alone.

Venus afflicted with the Moon will incline towards periodical ulcerations of the throat, and sage tea will remedy this.

Venus afflicted with the Sun by progression inclines to sore throat and watery discharges from the nostrils. A Taurus herb will be necessary.

Venus afflicted with Saturn inclines toward ague and chills, and a Martial and Taurus herb should be combined.

Venus afflicted with Jupiter inclines towards excesses, and a fruit fast will be best, combined with a Venus or Jupiter herb.

Venus afflicted with Uranus brings strange nervous disorders, sometimes induced by inoculations. Mercury and Taurus herbs will be necessary.

Venus afflicted with Neptune gives disorders of a neurotic type. A combination of Taurus and Aries herbs will be required, to cleanse and, at the same time, render the body more positive.

The Herbs of Gemini

The third house of the horoscope is ruled by Gemini and describes the arms and breathing power; and since it is the house of the thinking ability, it also describes the nervous system, for on the quality for our thoughts depends the health of the nervous system.

The Sun enters Gemini on May 21 and leaves it on June 21.

Mercury is the planetary ruler and those born when the Sun is in Gemini, especially during the morning hours, display the Mercurial characteristics of the message bearer and are usually quick and versatile thinkers.

The complaints of Gemini are bronchial affections, neuritis in the arms and shoulders, and nervous debility. Blood impurities and brain fevers are also Gemini complaints, the former resulting from insufficient breathing or foul atmosphere and the latter from lack of mental control or excessive study.

THE BEST KNOWN HERBS OF GEMINI ARE:

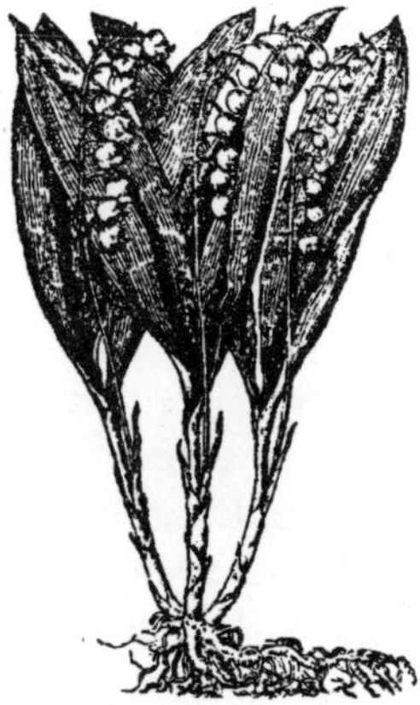

LILY OF THE VALLEY

LILY OF THE VALLEY is not so well known for its medicinal properties but it is useful in nervous disorders and the expressed juice will strengthen the eyes which are weakened through mental strain or study. When fright takes away the speech, this is restored by the flowers of this herb boiled in wine.

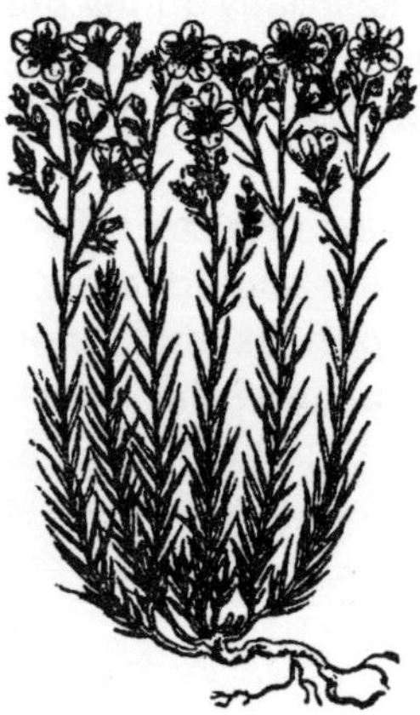

FLAX

FLAX or **LINSEED TEA** is well known since it is one of the oldest remedies for coughs, usually the method of preparation is to boil it with licorice and lemon. It is soothing to the bronchials and eaten raw is a fine laxative. The expressed oil, used externally, relieves asthma.

SKULLCAP is good for all complaints arising from nervous excitability, such as fits, convulsions, delirium tremens, St. Vitus' dance, neuritis, and neuralgia. A quart of water to one ounce makes it the required strength. It should be drunk at night, and in extreme cases every four hours during the day.

Parsley is used as a flavoring only, but is a nervine and blood purifier. It relieves inflamed eyes, when worry or study is the cause. As a tea, it's soothing and healing to people of Gemini type.

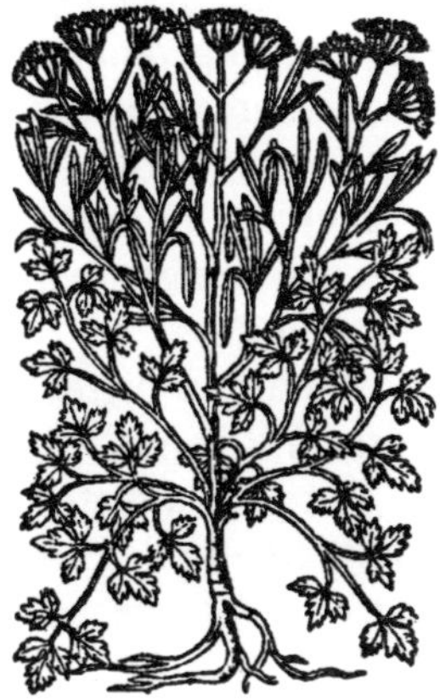

Parsley

Ferns, Meadowsweet, Caraway, and **Lavender** are under the rulership of Mercury and Gemini.

For Astrological Students

While each sign will give the predisposition to disease, interplanetary vibrations will give a more particular indication.

In the Gemini type, Mercury afflicted with Venus, by progression, has a powerful effect upon the mind, keying the nervous system to a high emotional pitch sometimes amounting to insanity. Any nervines except Valerian will help.

Mercury afflicted with Mars leads to nervous prostration, neuralgia and neuritis. The herbs of Mars will be necessary as a stimulant and tonic, as well as the nervines of Mercury.

Mercury afflicted with Jupiter leads to blood impurities. Jupiter herbs will be best.

Mercury afflicted with Saturn will require the harmonizing Venus herbs, as well as nervines.

Mercury afflicted with the Moon requires nervines and tonics.

Mercury afflicted with the Sun by progression affects eye sight, which will be helped by herbs of the Sun.

Mercury afflicted by Uranus causes mental worry and nervines are necessary.

Mercury afflicted with Neptune causes a chaotic mental condition and nervines, as well as tonics, are necessary.

The Herbs of Cancer

The fourth house of the horoscope is ruled by Cancer and as this house describes the stomach and mammary glands, so the complaints of Cancer are very closely connected with the stomach and breast.

The Sun enters Cancer about June 22 and leaves it about July 22. The Moon is the planetary ruler and those born while the Sun is passing through the sign are, like the Moon, reflective, changeable, orderly, adaptive yet defensive.

Just as the Moon reflects its surroundings so are its subjects easily influenced by and susceptible to their surroundings.

The complaints of Cancer are indigestion and all weaknesses of the breast, chest and stomach, cancerous growths, dropsy, asthma and pleurisy.

The herbs of the planetary ruler will often help, but as the Cancer subject is so negative when ailing, the more stimulating herbs of one of the other signs often should be used.

THE BEST KNOWN HERBS OF CANCER ARE:

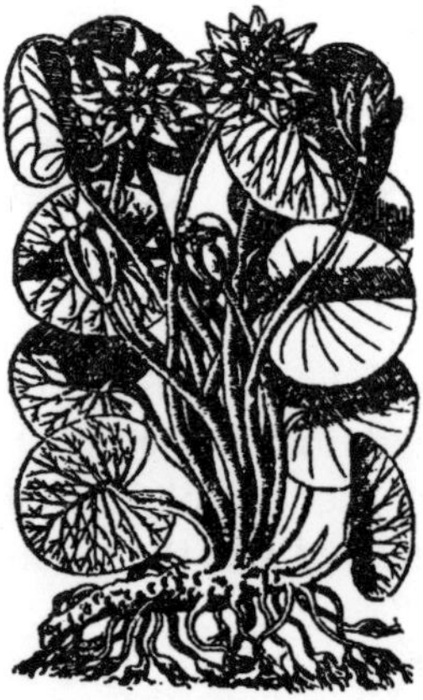

WATER LILY

WATER LILY is good for an ulcerated stomach but must be used carefully. It is most valuable as a wash for external ulcers. The juice from the flowers will remove freckles and sunburn.

DOG'S TOOTH VIOLET, its expressed juice is good for dropsy, the leaves are cooling and healing if placed on ulcerous growths. The root, simmered in milk will remove stomach worms and relieve an ulcerated stomach.

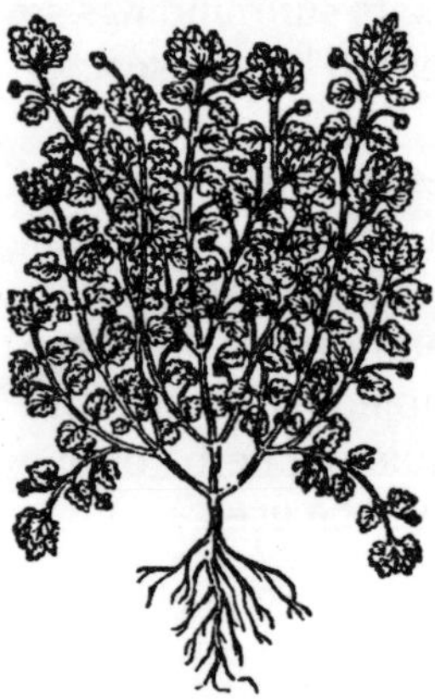

CHICKWEED

CHICKWEED, an ointment made from this is excellent for erysipelas. It enters largely into the herbal remedies for obesity. As a poultice it is good for ulcerous sores and as a tea it will relieve an ulcerated stomach.

Honeysuckle, one of the best remedies for stomach cramps, the leaves only being used.

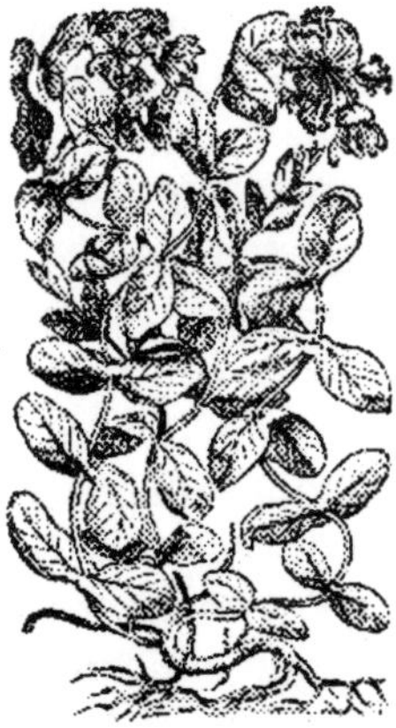

Honeysuckle

Lettuce is also a Cancer plant and its soothing sedative properties are well known.

For Astrological Students

The sign position and relationship of the Moon to other planets is very important in judging the Cancer predisposition to disease.

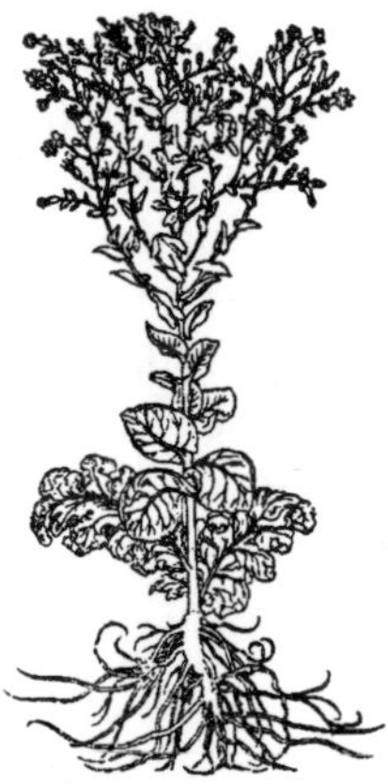

Lettuce

To give the inner meaning of each sign separately would take too much space here, but the sign and house indicate the prevailing thoughts and health depends on these.

Interplanetary vibrations intensify thought in various directions and lead to inharmony and ill health.

Moon afflicting Sun affects eyesight and leads to spasmodic affections and cramps. Cancer and Leo herbs should be combined.

Moon afflicting Venus inclines towards sagging of the inter-cellular tissues and cancer, dropsy and varicose veins often result.

Moon afflicting Mercury induces nervous disorders and Gemini or Virgo herbs will be best.

Moon afflicting Mars gives an overheated blood stream and the cooling Saturnine herbs or herbs of Venus should be used.

Moon afflicting Jupiter inclines towards impurities of the blood leading to boils, pimples, eruptive diseases. Sagittarius and Cancer herbs should be combined to combat this.

Moon afflicting Saturn gives chills and colds that require Martial tonics.

Moon afflicting Uranus inclines towards nervous disorders which can be overcome by nervines and tonics. Avoid the herbs of Mars as these are over-stimulating.

Moon afflicting Neptune will affect in a similar manner to Venus except that there is also a nervous or neurotic condition. The herbs of Mercury will help.

The Herbs of Leo

The fifth house of the horoscope, the house of children, speculation, education and pleasure, is ruled by Leo, and this sign governs the heart and arterial circulation.

The Sun enters Leo on July 23 and leaves it August 23. The Sun is the planetary ruler of the sign and those born in the morning during this period display the Sun characteristics of faith, optimism and the desire to rule and lead. Just as the Sun is the center of our universe, so they aim to be the center of their circle of acquaintances.

The complaints of Leo are heart affections, convulsions, pleurisy, palpitation, inflammatory fever, jaundice, sore eyes, cramp and spasms.

The herbs of Leo strengthen the eyes, equalize circulation, and relieve spasmodic affections.

THE MOST IMPORTANT OF THEM ARE:

WAKE ROBIN is a remedy for asthma, the root, bruised or pulverized is used, sweetened, with honey.

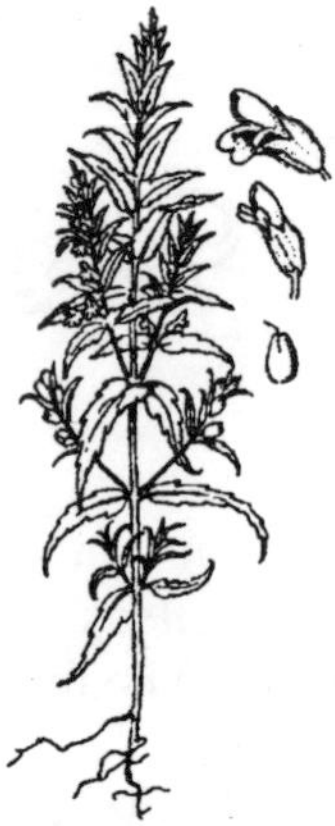

EYEBRIGHT

EYEBRIGHT is used as a wash for inflamed eyes. It may also be used internally and is good for earache, colds, coughs, and headache. If taken before breakfast, it is good for epilepsy.

MISTLETOE is a stimulant and tonic for a nervous heart. It is good for convulsive fits, palsy and vertigo.

MARIGOLD is a remedy for sore eyes, especially during measles. The juice is said to remove warts.

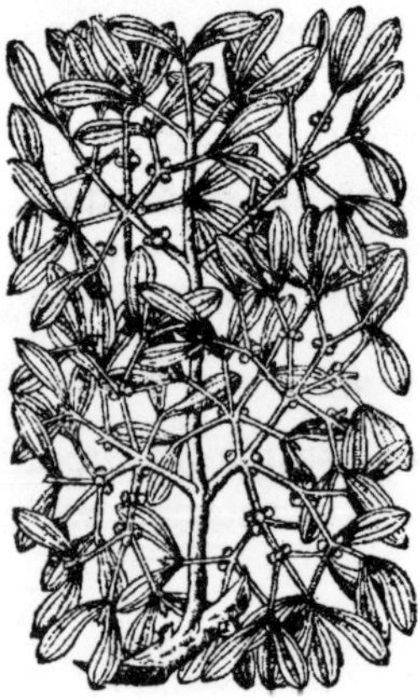

MISTLETOE

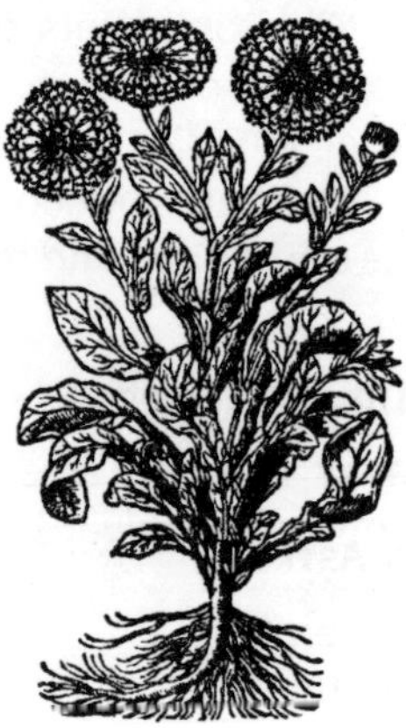

MARIGOLD

Walnuts are one of the finest Leo foods and should be added to every salad, fruit or vegetable.

St. John's Wort is one of the best remedies for asthma. Externally, it is used as an ointment for dispelling tumors.

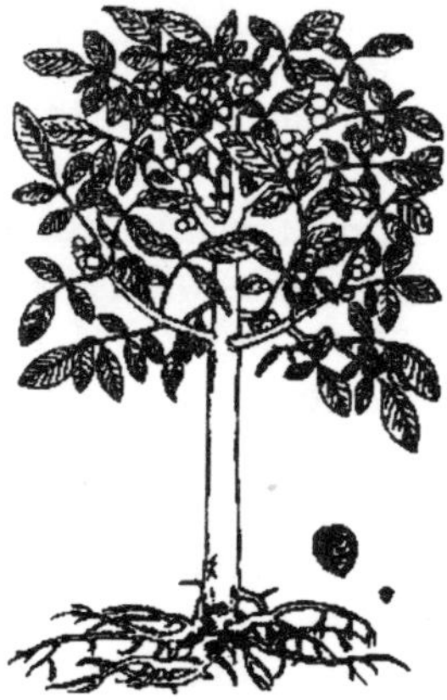

Walnuts

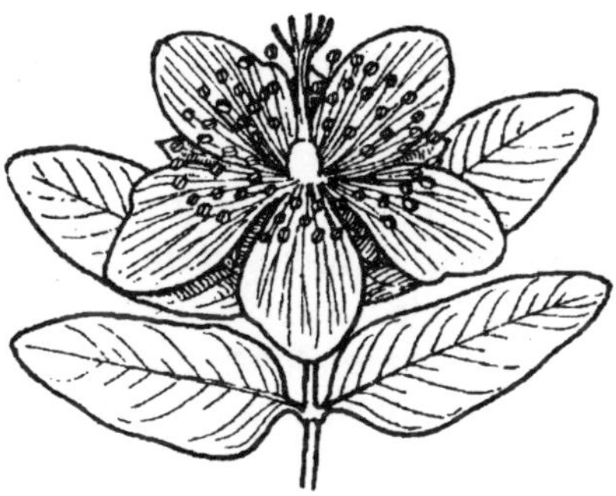

St. John's Wort

For Astrological Students

Interplanetary relationships between the Sun and other planets chiefly affected arterial circulation with its attendant evils.

Sun and Moon afflicted affects eyesight. Herbs of the Sun will give tone and strength.

Sun and Mercury by parallel or progression incline towards fear and nervous heart. Mercurial herbs will be best.

Sun and Venus by parallel or progression tend towards sluggish circulation. Stimulating Leo or Aries herbs will be best.

Sun and Mars overheat the blood, and the cooling Venus or Saturn herbs should be used to counteract.

Sun and Jupiter affect the liver and eyesight. Avoid all Martial herbs. Venus, Jupiter and Sun herbs and food will help. Appetite should be controlled, and frequent fasts may be necessary.

Sun and Saturn afflicted give gouty and rheumatic complaints, and sudorific herbs of Venus will be necessary.

Sun and Uranus afflicted give deep-seated complaints of the nervous system. Mercurial and Sun herbs will help.

Sun and Neptune afflicted affect the astral fluid. Tonics and nervines will be necessary.

Sun afflicted with the Moon's Nodes will act like Sun and Saturn.

The Herbs of Virgo

The sixth house of the horoscope, the house which governs voluntary service, is ruled by Virgo, the sign which governs liver, solar plexus and the intestines.

The Sun enters Virgo on August 23 and leaves it on September 23. Mercury is the planetary ruler and those born in the morning during this period, display the Mercurial characteristics of discrimination and love of scientific research, or, in less advanced types, criticism and fault finding.

The complaints of Virgo are dysentery, obstructions in the bowels, intestinal worms, colic gastritis, nervous disorders, and appendicitis. The organ mainly responsible for this is the liver, the physical seat of responsibility.

The herbs of Virgo must nourish the liver and educate it back to normal activity, soothe the nervous system, allay fear and heal the intestinal tract.

THE MOST COMMON VIRGO HERBS ARE:

SKULLCAP will tone the nervous system, and strengthen the solar plexus, the seat of fear.

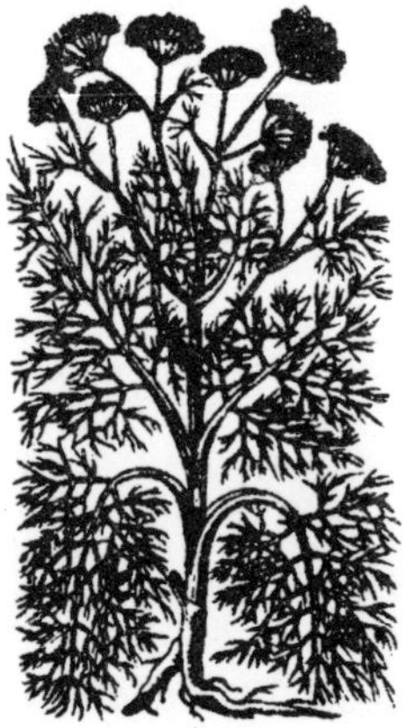

FENNEL

FENNEL will counteract flatulency.

MANDRAKE is a powerful liver cleanser, but should be used sparingly and with other herbs of a milder nature. It is one of the best agents, properly used, for cancerous conditions of the blood stream.

ENDIVE cools the liver and allays inflammation.

LICORICE sweetens the blood and reduces fever in the intestines.

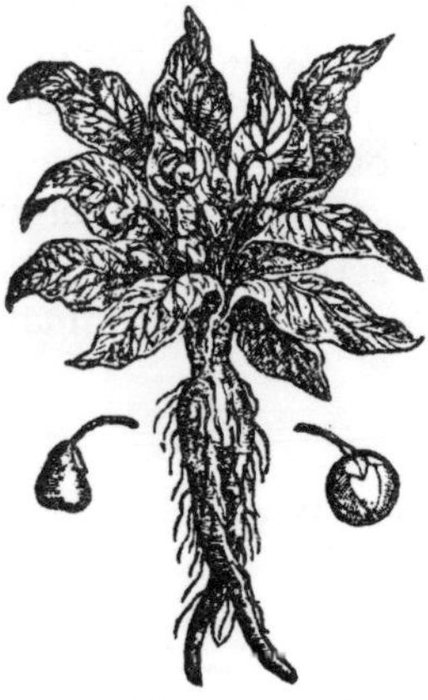

MANDRAKE

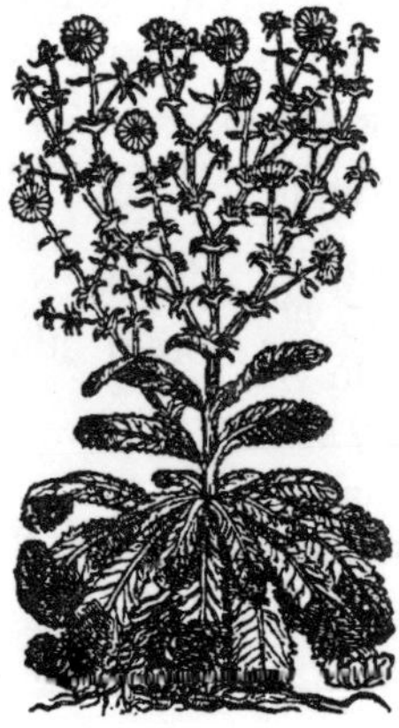

ENDIVE

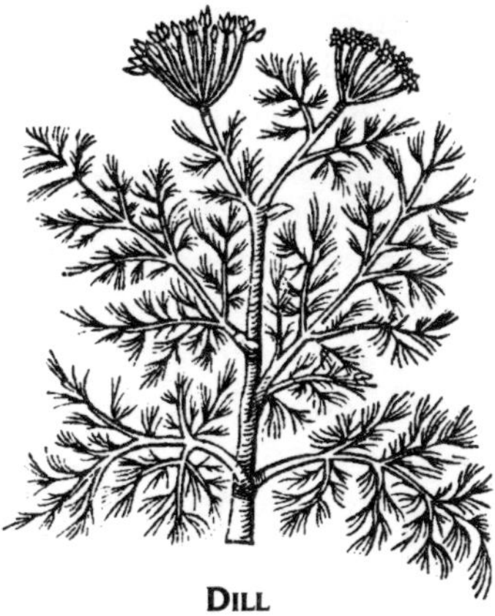

Dill

Dill will cleanse the digestive tract of ulcerations.

Pillory of the Wall removes obstructions of the liver. Added to marshmallow and made into an ointment it will cleanse and heal fistulas.

For Astrological Students

While each zodiacal sign gives a general idea of the part of the body likely to be affected, interplanetary vibrations give a more particular indication.

In Virgo subjects, the sign and aspects of Mercury as well as afflictions from the other Common signs, will give the history of liver disturbances, and on the healthy activity of the liver depends the health of the solar plexus and intestines, as well as the nervous system generally.

Mercury afflicted with Mars calls for Mercurial and Venus herbs. Liver tonics must be avoided until the over-acidity resulting from that planetary combination has been checked.

Mercury afflicted with the Sun requires the herbs of Leo to eliminate eye strain.

Mercury afflicted with the Moon can be helped by nervines and Cancer herbs.

Mercury afflicted with Jupiter requires the alternatives of Sagittarius and nervines of Virgo combined, but avoid the herbs of Mars.

Mercury afflicted with Saturn induces nervous strain and the soothing Venus herbs combined with nervines will help.

Mercury afflicted with Uranus inclines towards extreme nervous affections. Nervines and demulcents should be combined.

Mercury afflicted with Venus and Neptune excites the nervous system. Venus and Mercury herbs give relief.

Whenever Mercury is afflicted, the nerve fluids are affected and the various nerve centers of the body are congested.

Nervines must be used as well as laxatives, for nervines by themselves tend towards constipating he bowels.

Nervines and laxatives can be combined without one reducing the effect of the other.

The Herbs of Libra

The seventh house of the horoscope, the house of marriage and business partners, is ruled by Libra, the sign which governs the kidneys, the seat of domestic harmony.

The Sun enters Libra September 23 and leaves it October 23. Those born in the morning during this period display the Venus-Libra characteristics of desiring the association of others. In less advanced types partnerships are quickly formed and broken, approbativeness being the strongest trait.

The complaints of Libra are kidney stones, pains in the back, inflammation of the kidneys and bladder, general debility. Libra is one of the most important signs in the horoscope for on this, wherever it is placed, depends our poise and balance.

When there are afflictions from the sign Libra, the blood loses its alkaline properties and a physical condition known as over-acidity results. This affects the stomach causing flatulency, affects the sweat glands, causing unpleasant body odors, weakens the kidneys leading to various forms of kidney disease and finally affects the lower brain leading to hallucinations and insanity.

The herbs of Libra then must tone the kidneys, keep the pores of the skin active that the daily load of carbonaceous waste material may be lessened and restore the sodium phosphate, the mineral salt which helps to maintain the balance between acids and alkalis.

Some of the herbs of Libra are to be found in every district where human life is possible.

THE FOLLOWING HERBS ARE THE MOST COMMON:

VIOLET is recognized as a remedy for internal and external cancer, a disease condition which always indicates lack of phosphates. It has a cooling effect on the kidneys and is a remedy for scalding urine.

BAYBERRY is a kidney tonic, but should be used only with the milder herbs.

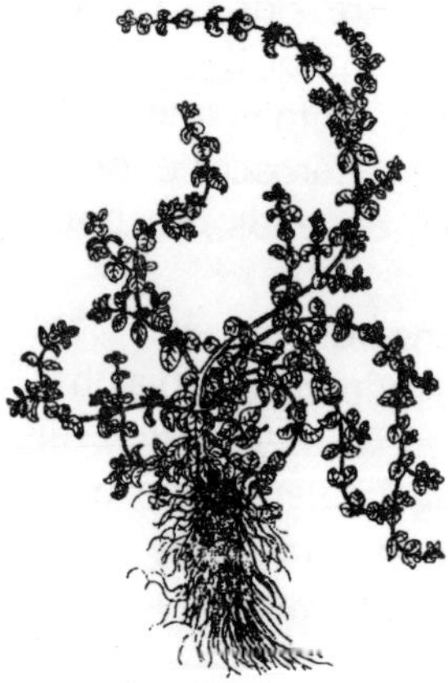

PENNYROYAL

THYME is excellent for headaches and giddiness arising from nervous kidneys.

PENNYROYAL is soothing and warming. Many mothers use a weak tea of this herb for feverish, teething babies.

ARCHANGEL opens the pores of the skin.

FEVERFEW will strengthen and cleanse the kidneys.

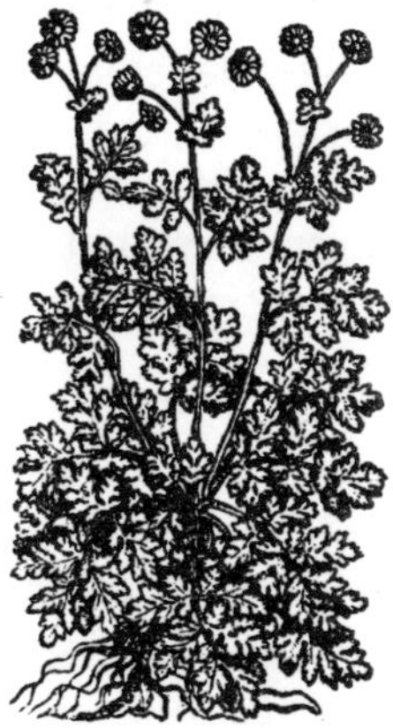

FEVERFEW

SILVERWEED is useful where there is over-activity of the kidneys, but this should be used cautiously and combined with a herb of an emollient nature.

CATMINT is similar to Pennyroyal and Feverfew in its action.

BURDOCK may be safely used in all forms of kidney weakness.

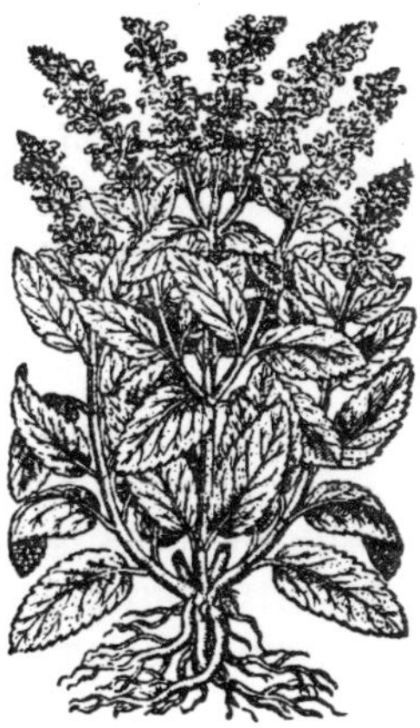

CATMINT

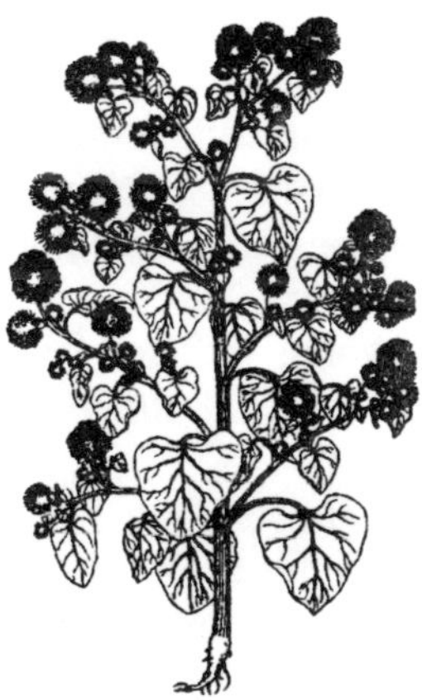

BURDOCK

For Astrological Students

Interplanetary vibrations are very important in considering the health condition of the Libra type. We have here involved the planets of Venus, Saturn, Mars and the Moon, which are intimately associated with home and honor, and on these depend the healthy activity of the kidneys.

Venus afflicted with Mars increases sensitivity to criticism, which leads to nervous breakdowns and sometimes depravity in various forms. The herbs of Mars or Venus will help. Saturn's herbs may be used alone.

Venus afflicted with Mercury often weakens the moral fibre. Mercurial herbs will give tone to the nerves.

Venus afflicted with the Moon affects the glandular system. The tonics of Mars with the sudorifics of Venus will help.

Venus afflicted with the Sun by progression causes chills. Sun herbs will assist.

Venus afflicted by Saturn affects sex organs, often leading to moral depravity. Saturnine herbs will be most useful in reducing inflammatory conditions.

Venus afflicted by Uranus is similar in effect to Mercurial afflictions. Nervines will be most useful.

Venus afflicted with Neptune disturbs the astral fluids and so leads to distorted imagination. Mars and Sun herbs will stimulate. Venus herbs are also necessary.

The Herbs of Scorpio

The eighth house of the horoscope, the house of possessions of partners, is ruled by Scorpio, and this sign governs the generative organs.

The Sun enters Scorpio on October 23 and leaves it November 22. Mars is the planetary ruler and those born in the morning during this period display the Martial characteristics of self-confidence, energy and activity and, in less evolved types, pride, vanity and passion.

The complaints of Scorpio are secret diseases connected with the generative organs, ruptures, piles, uterine troubles, catarrh of the bladder, etc.

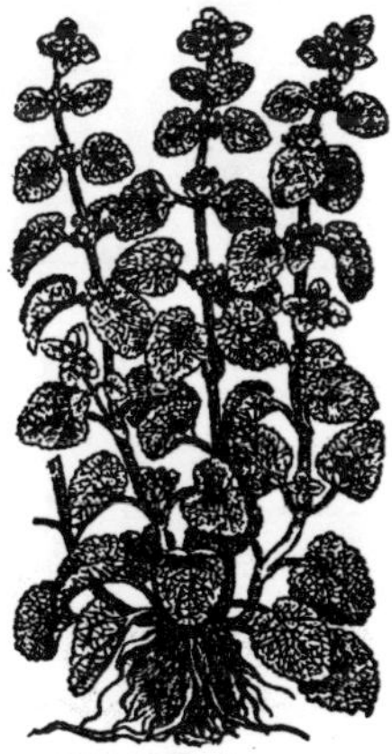
HOREHOUND

The herbs of Scorpio are cleansing and antiseptic, forcing impurities to leave the body by natural channels—the bladder, skin, and intestines.

The best known herbs of Scorpio are **HOREHOUND, BLACKBERRY LEAVES,**

BLESSED THISTLE, LEEK, HORSERADISH, TOAD-FLAX, WORMWOOD, and **SARSAPARILLA,** all of which have antiseptic, healing properties, which stimulate the glandular system so it can throw off the poisonous wastes which may otherwise accumulate in the throat, bladder or generative organs, causing serious inflammatory disorders.

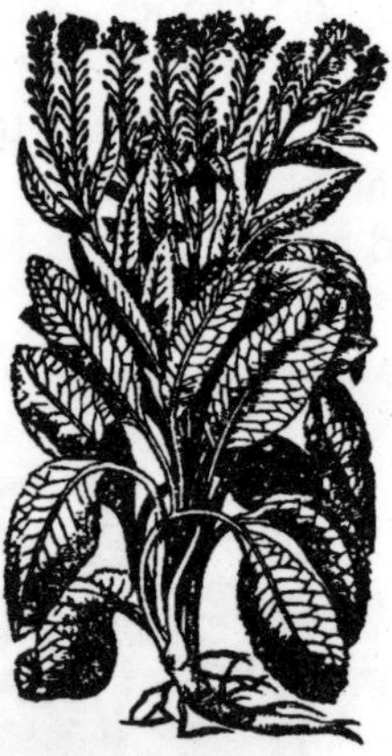

HORSERADISH

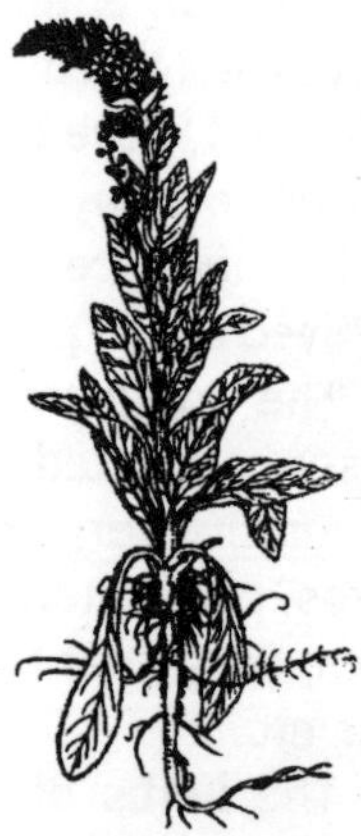

TOAD-FLAX

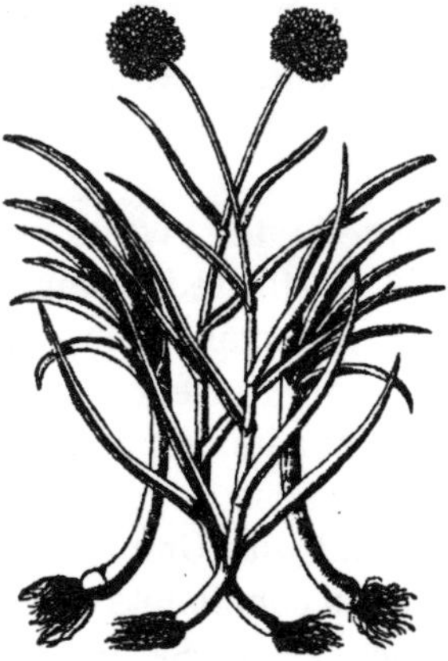

LEEK

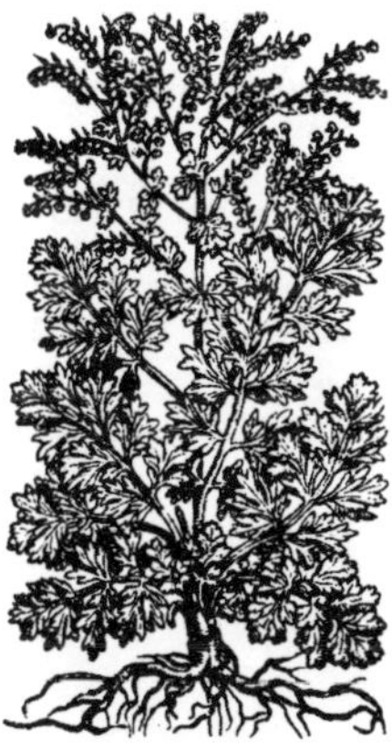

WORMWOOD

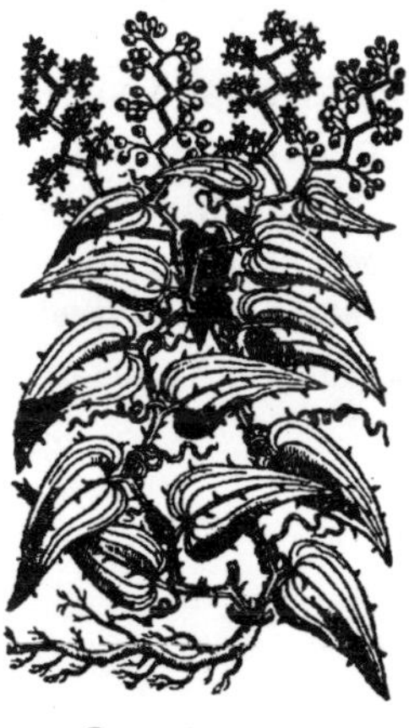

SARSAPARILLA

For Astrological Students

The position and aspects of Mars should be carefully noted in the health study of the Scorpio type.

Mars elevated often gives a very strong constitution, but if afflicted, complaints are very sudden, deep-seated and complicated.

Mars afflicted with Neptune inclines towards neurotic thoughts and actions. Cooling Saturnine herbs will be best.

Mars afflicted with Uranus inclines towards nervous, feverish complaints. Use Gemini herbs.

Mars afflicted with Saturn gives rheumatic tendencies. Venus herbs will give best results.

Mars afflicted with Venus is similar to affliction with Neptune.

Mars afflicted with Mercury produces nervous disorders and should be treated with Martial and Mercurial herbs.

Mars afflicted with the Sun overheats the blood and Leo and Venus herbs will remedy.

Mars afflicted with the Moon will be similar in effect to Venus and Neptune.

The Herbs of Sagittarius

The ninth house of the horoscope, the house of philosophy, religion, law and long journeys, is ruled by Sagittarius, and this sign governs the thighs, the organs of locomotion.

The Sun enters Sagittarius on November 22 and leaves it December 21. Those born in the morning during this period display the optimistic characteristics of Jupiter and the desire to take chances in seeking new worlds to conquer, as well as new philosophies of life.

The complaints of Sagittarius are accidents through haste and violent exercise; feverish complaints through excesses and overheated blood, rheumatism and neuritis in the lower limbs and, since Jupiter endows many of its subjects with an inordinate amount of pride—and goiter is a disease of injured pride or humiliation—goiter may be classed as a Sagittarius complaint.

Some forms of cancer may also be classed as Sagittarius complaints, especially cancer of the liver and intestines; but where this is the case it will be found that Jupiter is afflicted in one of the Common signs.

The herbs of Sagittarius cool the blood, reduce fever and heal.

THE MOST IMPORTANT OF THEM ARE:

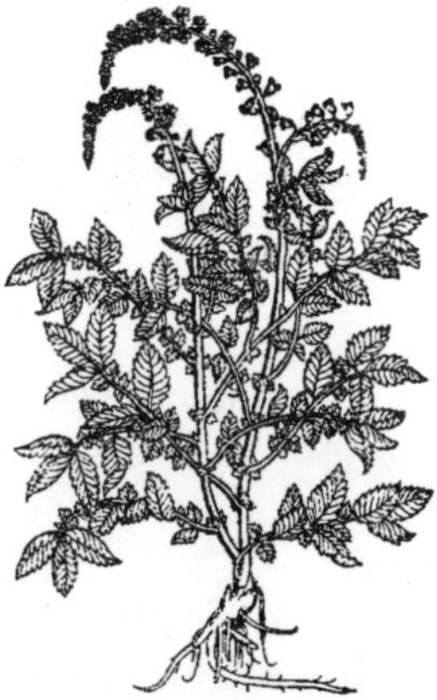

AGRIMONY

AGRIMONY, which will allay fever and tone the liver.

BURDOCK, which is cooling and purifying to the blood stream.

CHICORY is good for liver impurities, which result from overheated blood.

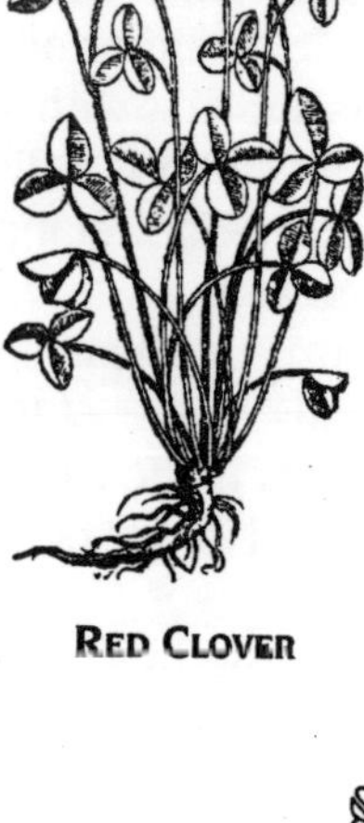

RED CLOVER

RED CLOVER, is one of the most efficacious remedies for goiter.

PODOPHYLLUM or **MAY APPLE** has no equal in acting in and through the tissues, cleansing, healing and purifying. It is one of the best herbs for internal cancer.

Dandelion is a member of the chicory family, and is of value in cleansing the over-heated blood stream.

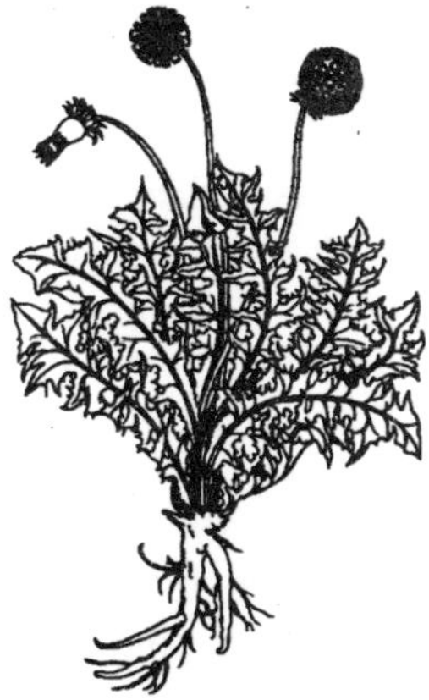

Dandelion

Oak is a fine astringents and was used by many herbalists during small-pox epidemics as a preventative. The bark is boiled and the body bathed with the liquid. It is also used as a cure for goiter, the method is to soak a cloth in an oak bark solution each evening and wrap it around the throat, covering with a dry cloth.

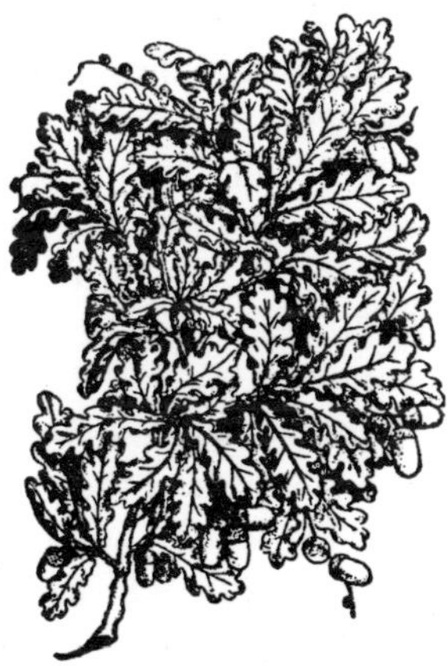

Oak

For Astrological Students

Jupiter, the ruler of Sagittarius, must be carefully studied as the house and sign for correct diagnosis of disease. For instance, Jupiter afflicted with the Moon will, in some cases, lead to obesity and, in others, lack of appetite.

Jupiter afflicted with Neptune or Venus is a frequent forerunner of goiter, and Jupiter herbs will relieve.

Jupiter afflicted with Saturn leads to sluggish action of the blood, ending in nervous prostration, neuritis, and rheumatism, Nervines combined with the herbs of Sagittarius should be used.

Jupiter adverse with Mercury causes headaches, dizziness and sometimes congestion of the brain. Nervines and Jupiter herbs should be used here.

Jupiter in affliction with the Sun sometimes leads to apoplexy, palpitation of the heart and the loss of sight in one eye, if in Fixed signs. Jupiter herbs will be best but living must be abstemious.

Jupiter afflicted with Mars gives impure blood, diseases of the liver, liability to burns and accidents. Martial herbs should be used.

Jupiter afflicted with Uranus affects the nervous system. Jupiter and Gemini herbs should be used.

The Herbs of Capricorn

The tenth house of the horoscope is ruled by Capricorn and describes the knees, bone structure, and skin.

The Sun enters Capricorn on the 22 of December and leaves it on the 20 of January.

Saturn is the planetary ruler and those born when the Sun is in Capricorn, especially during the morning hours, will display the Saturnine characteristics of ambition, diplomacy and tact, or secretiveness and cunning.

The complaints of Capricorn are rheumatism of the knees and lower limbs, skin diseases, fractures, weak knees, leprosy, ruptures, corns, rickets, and warts.

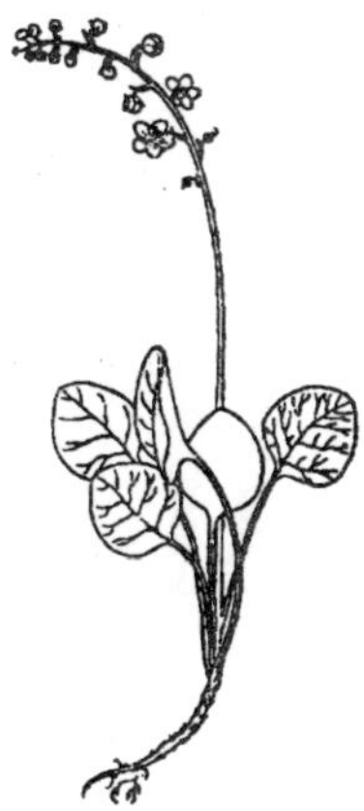

WINTERGREEN

THE BEST KNOWN HERBS OF CAPRICORN ARE:

WINTERGREEN is a remedy for rheumatism in the joints.

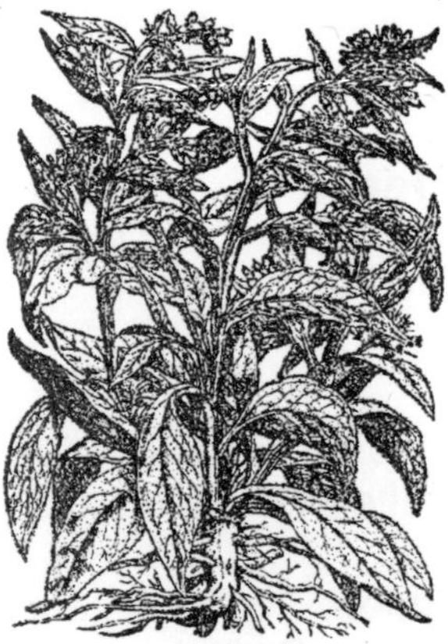

COMFREY

COMFREY ROOT is an excellent remedy for ruptures and skin complaints. It should be grown in every garden as it is more efficacious if used fresh. Used externally, the leaves or the expressed juice will reduce swellings and heal ruptures. An ointment made from the green root will cure warts.

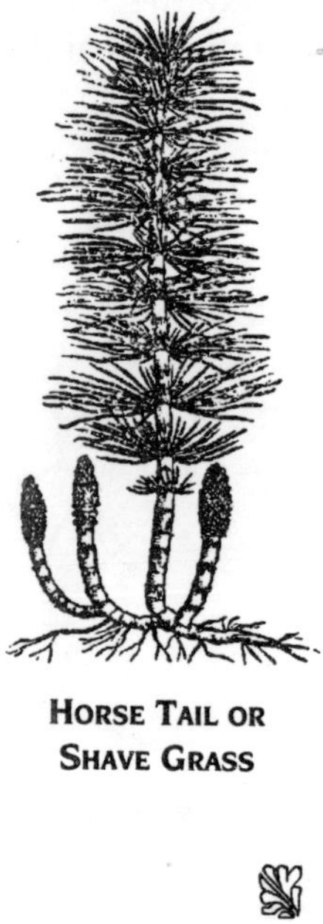

HORSE TAIL OR SHAVE GRASS

HORSE TAIL or **SHAVE GRASS** will stop internal hemorrhages and an ointment made from it will relieve inflammatory sores.

THUJA is one of the best remedies for warts on any part of the body. It will relieve sore eyes and sometimes take away cataracts.

Fumitory and **Thyme** are also Capricorn herbs.

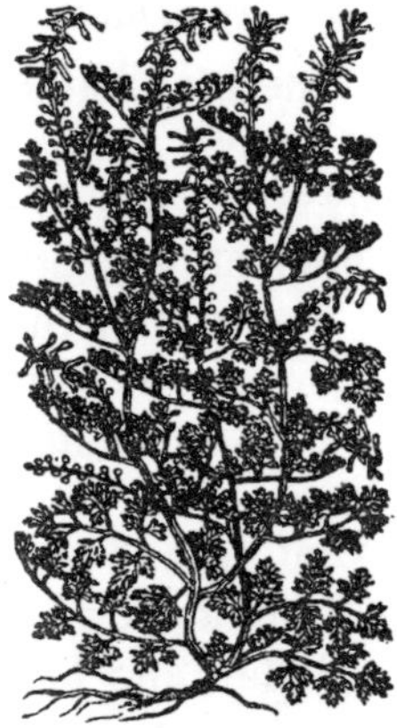

Fumitory

Knot Grass dissolves phlegm, checks bleeding from the mouth and nose and the expressed juice heals external wounds. It hastens the healing of broken joints and ruptures and the juice will stop running ears.

Slippery Elm is a fine food and medicine. It is cooling, healing, and soothing for the entire digestive tract. It is the best and most nutritious baby food as it strengthens the bone structure and allays inflammatory tendencies. It should be kept in every household.

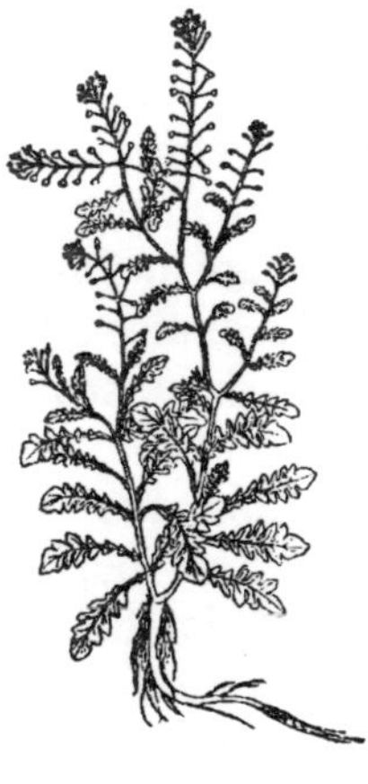

Shepherd's Purse

Shepherd's Purse is similar in effect to Knot Grass.

For Astrological Students

The stimulating herbs of Mars are efficacious for many Capricorn complaints, but interplanetary action will sometimes indicate a need for a combination of other herbs.

Saturn and the Sun afflicted cause palpitation of the heart, paralysis, sore eyes, and cataracts. Leo herbs are best, combined with Slippery Elm.

Saturn and Jupiter afflicted incline towards ruptures and Comfrey Root will be best.

Saturn and Mars also incline towards ruptures, rheumatism, mucous in the throat and deafness. Martial herbs combined with Slippery Elm should be used.

Saturn and the Moon afflicted induce colds and flatulence complaints. Martial herbs will be best.

Saturn and Mercury induce nervous debility and affect the solar plexus. the herbs of the Sun and Mercury will give the best results.

Saturn and Venus incline towards diseases of the generative organs and lingering inflammatory and skin diseases. Slippery Elm and Venusian or Martial herbs should be used.

Saturn and Uranus seem to be sudden in their action, but they give evidence of deep-seated complaints involving the nervous and renal system. These require stimulating and nervine herbs. Sage and Skullcap are beneficial.

The Herbs of Aquarius

The eleventh house of the horoscope is ruled by Aquarius and describes the condition of the calf and ankles. Aquarius also affects the blood stream through sympathy with Leo, its opposite sign, which rules the arterial circulation.

The Sun enters Aquarius about the 20 of January and leaves it on February 19.

Uranus is the planetary ruler and those born when the Sun is in Aquarius, especially during the morning hours, display the Uranian characteristics of eccentricity and willfulness, until they recognize their life work and are attached to either a person or a cause.

Restriction in any form is irritating to the Aquarian, yet, paradoxical as it may seem, inwardly they crave discipline.

This probably accounts for so many of them entering some form of government service, especially where a uniform is worn, such as in the army, navy, hospitals, asylums or prisons.

Later in life they recognize that self-discipline is the only real discipline. They they realize that physical and mental control result in a healthy body.

The complaints of Aquarius are cramps in the calf of the leg, milk leg, rheumatic fever, blood impurities and paralysis. Since the sign is opposite Leo, the sun sign which rules one eye—the right in a man and left in a woman—the eyes are often affected.

The best known herbs of Aquarius are:

Valerian and **Lady's Slipper**. These may be used in hysteria, and delirium, as they quiet the nerves, allays pain and promotes sleep. One quart of water is used to one ounce of the herb powdered. One of the worst cases we have known of epilepsy was cured by the use of this herb, but it should be used carefully as, in some cases, it over-stimulates the brain, thus increasing rather than decreasing the trouble.

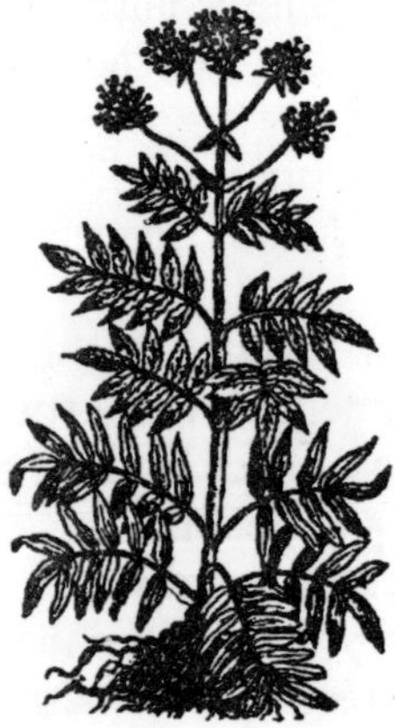

Valerian

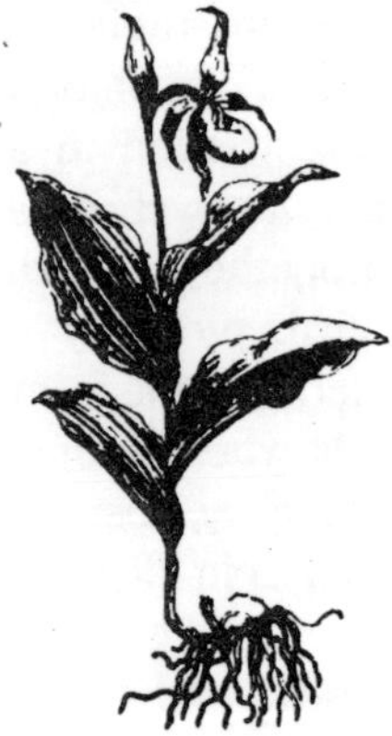

Lady's Slipper

SOUTHERNWOOD, popularly known as Old Man, is a remedy for hysteria.

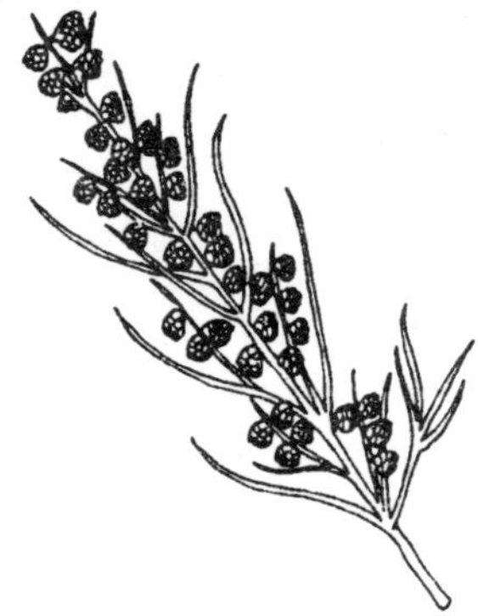

SOUTHERNWOOD

The herbs of Leo are a great help in Aquarian complaints, especially in removing the cause of hysteria and cramp.

SNAKE ROOT, also known as **SPOTTED PLANTAIN**, is most useful as a wash for inflamed eyes, although it may be used internally and will remedy cramps in the legs.

FOR ASTROLOGICAL STUDENTS

While each sign will give an idea of the predisposition to disease, the interplanetary vibrations give a more particular indication.

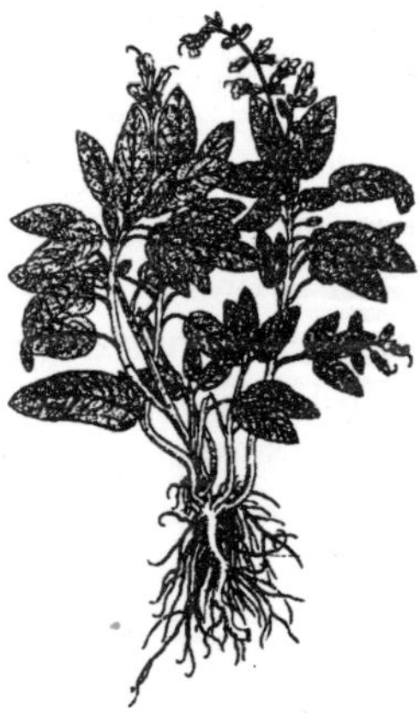

SAGE

In the Aquarian, Uranus afflicted with Mercury inclines to mental disorders and confusion. Such nervines as Valerian, in small doses, will give relief in young people.

There is usually, however, a deep-seated cause when this planetary combination makes itself felt in later life, usually traceable to sex abuse. In mild cases hallucination or obsession will be noticed, but in advanced cases, insanity requiring restraint will result.

To overcome this condition, the whole chart must be examined and the habits examined. Harmonizing Venus herbs will help. Stimulating Martial herbs sometimes do good, but more often harm and the herbs of Uranus will help to induce restful sleep.

It is always necessary to see that the liver is active, as well as the intestines regular, before giving herbs of a nervine nature, for poisons from the intestinal tract merely intensity the complaint.

Uranus afflicted with Venus leads to sexual excesses owing to the magnetic stimulation through this planetary combination. Southernwood is one of the best tonics for women and sage tea for men where over-stimulation leads to neurotic thoughts.Uranus afflicted with Mars leads to blood impurities through heat and impulsive thought and action. Uranian and Jupiter herbs will help. Saturnine herbs will cool the blood stream and check any tendency towards apoplexy.

Uranus afflicted with Jupiter leads to blood impurities, and cooling laxative Jupiter herbs will be best.

Uranus afflicted with the Sun will induce cramps, nervous and hysterical conditions. Uranian and Sun herbs combined will give relief.

Uranus afflicted with the Moon causes hysteria, nervous complaints, weakened eyesight. Uranian herbs combined with those under the Moon should be used.

Uranus afflicted with Saturn induces cold, rheumatic, and nervous disorders. The stimulating herbs of Mars will be useful here.

Uranus afflicted with Neptune will have a similar effect to the Venus and Mercurial afflictions and the same remedies apply.

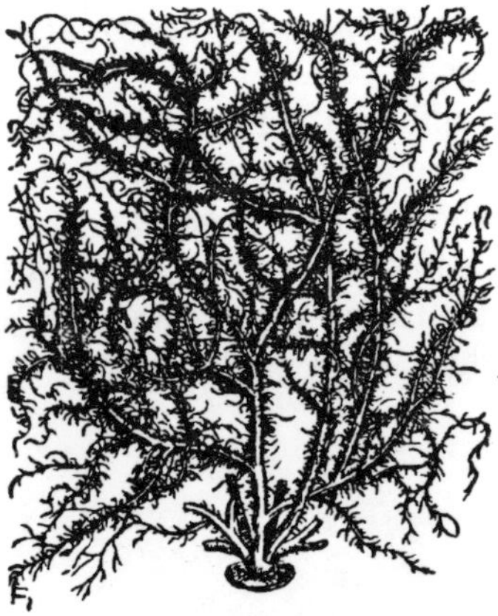

BRANCHED MOSS

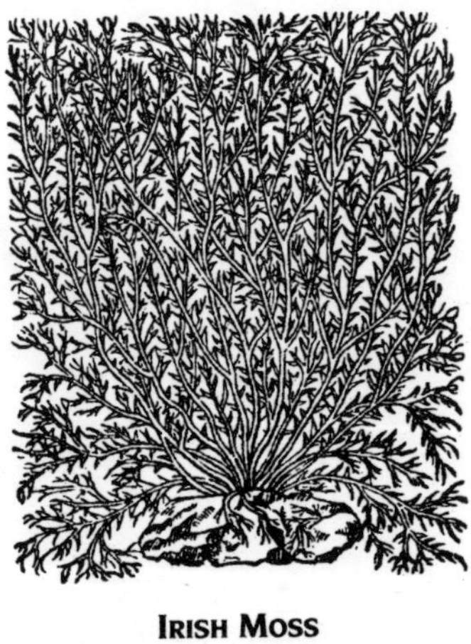

IRISH MOSS

The Herbs of Pisces

The twelfth house of the horoscope is ruled by Pisces and, since this describes the condition of the feet, it follows that complaints of Pisces are primarily complaints of the feet and toes.

The Sun enters Pisces on February 19 and leaves it on March 20. Neptune is the planetary ruler of Pisces, so those born while the Sun is passing through the sign display the Neptunian characteristics of pathos, winsomeness, and sympathy—or selfishness and cunning—according to the degree of their development.

The complaints of Pisces are gout, boils, ulcers, abscesses, corns, bunions, enlarged feet, lameness, etc., arising from cold and moisture.

The herbs of the planetary ruler, Neptune, will help, but Pisces is a negative sign, so the stimulating Martial herbs are often necessary to inspire the courage which the sick Pisces subject often lacks.

Pisces has rulership over all sea-weeds, sea-water mosses, and native water plants.

Irish Moss is a valuable Pisces herb. It is often called Consumptive's Moss because it relieves consumption. It should be soaked in water for twenty-four hours, then boiled in either milk or water.

If boiled in milk it can be used as a porridge. If boiled in water, add fruit juice and allow to set. It makes an excellent and nourishing invalid's jelly.

Most children relish Irish Moss if it is properly prepared, but for those who dislike it and cannot be persuaded to eat it as a porridge or jelly, it can be added to soups, where it is not noticed.

It contains iron and iodine in the only form in which these can be assimilated by the body.

An enterprising firm in the United States reduced the moss to a powder and sold it at a good profit under the name of Sea Lettuce—a suitable name, as it has the virtues of the lettuce plus the tonic qualities peculiar to itself.

If it is used persistently, Irish Moss will relieve practically every Pisces complaint and children raised upon it—for it is an economical food—will not be consumptive or goiter subjects.

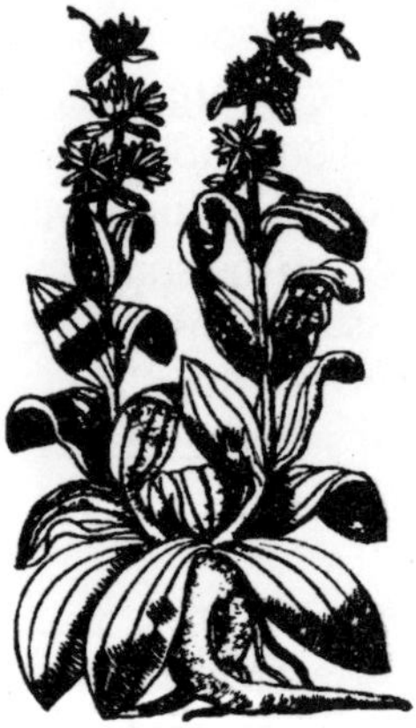

GENTIAN

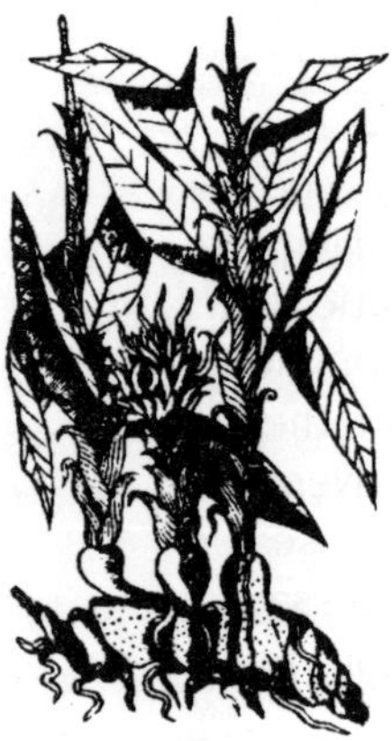

GINGER

FOR ASTROLOGICAL STUDENTS

In Pisces subjects, if Neptune and Mercury are afflicted, hallucinations are common and a Martial nervine is necessary, as well as a Neptunian herb. **CAYENNE**, **HOPS**, **GENTIAN**, or **GINGER**, added to **IRISH MOSS** will provide a remedy.

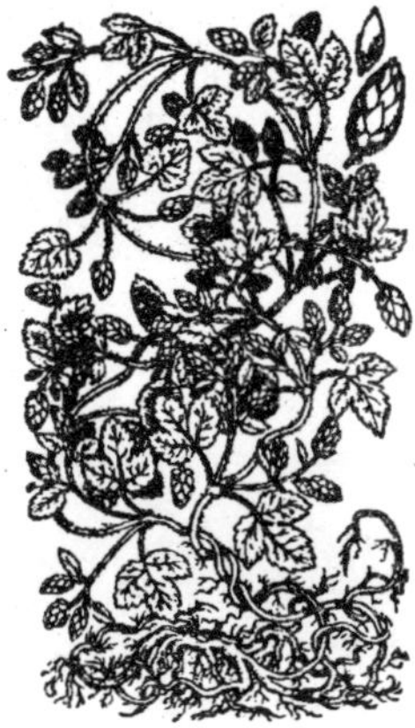

HOPS

Neptune and Venus incline to moral laxity, or afflictions of the generative organs. Irish Moss added to a Venus herb will remedy this.

Neptune and Jupiter afflicted create blood impurities so, for a remedy, add the Moss to a Jupiter herb.

Neptune and the Sun afflicted causes mental and emotional disturbances, and a Sun herb must be added to the moss to effect a cure.

Neptune and Saturn produce cold and rheumatic diseases, which can be overcome by the stimulating Martial herbs used in conjunction with the herbs.

Neptune and Mars incline towards emotional excesses and, in such cases, a blood purifier is necessary, such as **BLOOD-ROOT** or **SARSAPARILLA**, Scorpian herbs.

The part of the body most liable to affliction will be the part governed by the rising sign and the sign of its planetary ruler. Signs containing planets which form aspects with the planetary ruler of the ascendant must also be considered.

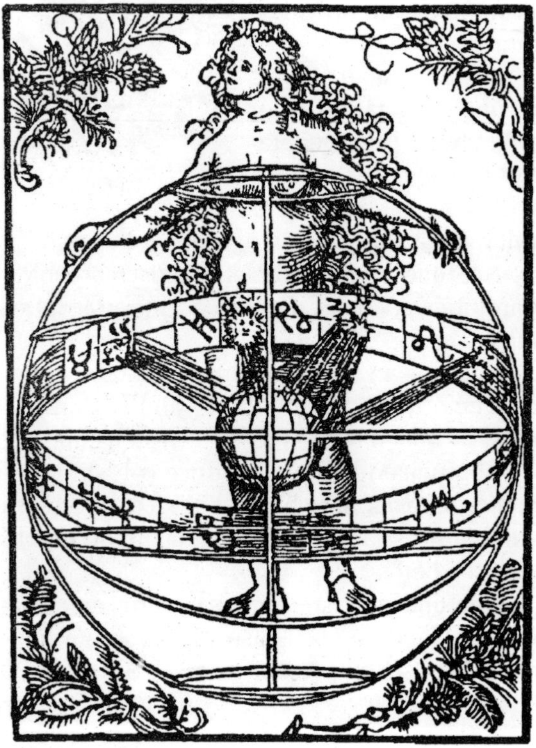

SECTION THREE:
HEALTH AND THE SUN SIGNS

BY ADA MUIR

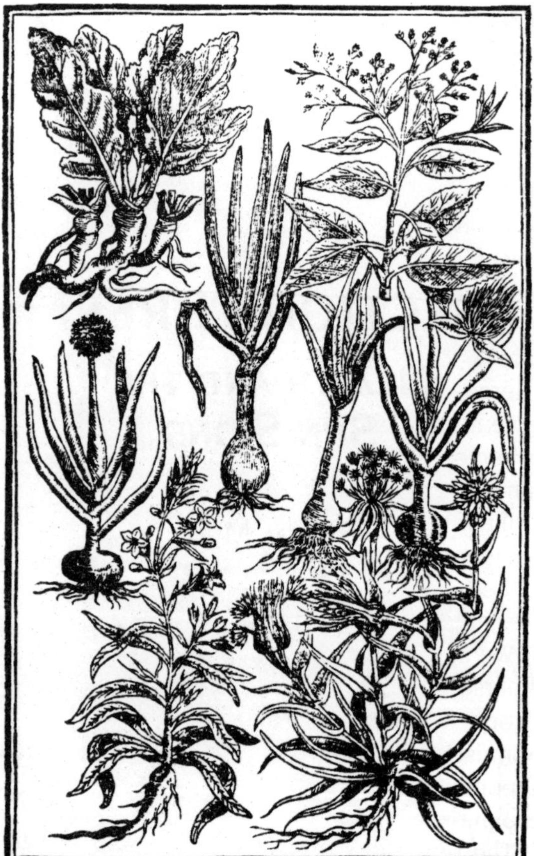

Introduction

Time was when every doctor was also an astrologer, for a knowledge of astrology was considered the only means of diagnosis and the means whereby a cure could be found.

But as the medical profession degenerated from a "calling" to a "profession," and people entered its ranks less from the Divine urge to serve humanity than from the desire to enter a respectable profession, astrology was dropped from the curriculum.

If astrology is to advance as a science, astrologers must demonstrate its utility, and there is no better or more useful field for this than in stressing it as an exact means of diagnosis.

We may study astrology from the standpoint of personal success and centralize our efforts on second, sixth, and tenth house affairs, but back we must come to the vitality—how will the body respond to the struggle for material success and recognition.

The triangle which rules those departments represented by second, sixth, and tenth houses will give us the physical reaction. It will give us the means which must be taken for constant recuperation, if material failure is not to result.

We may feel the urge for self-expression along mental lines and seek our field of work through first, fifth, and ninth houses. But we can only give of our best in creative idealism by recognizing the needs of the body. Unless the body is healthy, that which is created is tainted with disease even at its dawn.

This book cannot tell all that is known of the relationship between health and astrology. It is introductory and suggestive rather than conclusive, and is published to meet the desires of those who are seeking health through a knowledge of planetary vibrations.

Medicinal Astrology

Biochemists have discovered that certain mineral salts are necessary for the healthy activity of the human body. Astrologers go further and correlate these salts with the signs of the zodiac. The subject, however, has rarely been brought to its logical conclusion, for not only is it imperative to be able to tell why these salts are necessary but it is also essential to be able to tell when they are necessary.

By an analysis of the birth chart of the individual we may know the predisposition towards cell salt deficiency. This is so since the first and sixth houses indicate the greatest possibility of health strain—the first as being the most intensely personal house and the sixth as being the weakest from the physical standpoint. The sign in which the Sun is placed at birth will also tell of a special cell salt need, according to its relative position with regard to the other planets.

The cell salts of the zodiac are to be found in plant and vegetable life, since plants and vegetables absorb these salts from the soil. If our diet consists of fruit and vegetables, we are building into our system the cell salts necessary. But there are times when Nature makes a greater demand on some one cell salt than on another. These times and cell salts are indicated in the passage of the Moon through the sign of the zodiac.

It must be distinctly borne in mind that to partake of one or even a dozen of the cell salts will not necessarily produce health, although it may relieve a given situation. The cell salts cannot heal. It is essential that we know the spiritual essence of which the cell salt is the material expression and in seeking that state of spirituality volatilize the cell salt to its highest potency.

With the aid of the Sun, the plants have gathered the minerals from the soil in such a manner that we do not recognize them except by analysis. But we must go further than the plant and through our understanding of thought vibration, raise the mineral to its spiritual expression.

Many who have tried this method of healing have found themselves apparently worse a few days after commencing the treatment. They thereupon have denounced the system as being of no value, failing to understand that the physical suffering they experienced was due to the inability of the body to respond as quickly as the mind to the higher vibrations.

The great value of medicinal astrology lies in the fact that it enables the astrologer to gently lead the patient to an understanding of the thought vibration of the different signs of the zodiac and to a knowledge of the twelve gates of cosmic consciousness through which all must pass in their struggle toward God-consciousness. It is only through comprehension of cosmic consciousness and a sincere desire to contact its highest expression that we may experience health mentally, morally, and spiritually.

During each 28 years of our lives, in the progression of the Moon through the twelve signs of the zodiac, we have felt the different thought influences of each sign. The Moon takes approximately 28 months in its passage through each sign in the progressed horoscope, and each month will bring some variation in the mental outlook. But the variation is far greater in the passage of the Moon from sign to sign.

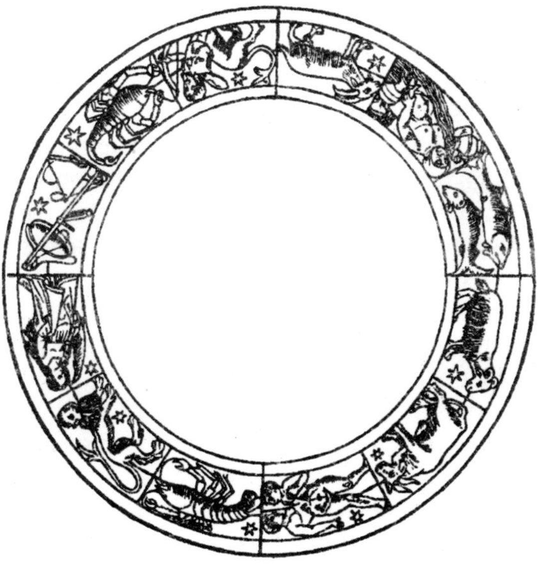

These variations of mental outlook bring experiences, the cream of which are added to the ego, represented by the Sun in the chart, and will be used to enrich the personal horoscope of the future.

Discordant vibrations between the Moon and other planets draw upon the vitality as shown by the Sun. Then the body is unable to utilize the necessary cell salt until there is a mental readjustment.

So it becomes necessary to understand the nature of the Sun sign and the function of its corresponding cell salt.

It becomes necessary to see ourselves face to face so we may know wherein we fail. We need the science of astrology to inform us to what extent we are in tune with the Infinite.

The body will inform us when all is not well and an analysis of the birth chart will inform us why all is not well.

In the following pages we have stressed the Sun sign as an important factor in health preservation for the Sun represents our center. The true secret of life is to find our center and to radiate from it.

We have purposely pointed out the mental condition accompanying the physical weakness and that self-cure is the only cure, but that self-analysis should precede an attempt at self-cure.

The man or woman whose blood is in an anemic condition through lack of iron has received a blow to courage in some form or other, and the iron in the blood cannot be restored by the

Pisces cell salt (sulfate of iron) until there is that mental readjustment that allows them to view every experience from the lessons that may be learned, for Pisces symbolizes self-surrender.

The brain fogged from over-work or miscarriage of plans will not be restored by the Aries cell salt (potassium phosphate) until there is thorough mental relaxation to equalize the circulation through the congested brain cells.

Intellectual activity driven by the will distorts mental vision. But thought-control resulting in constructive idealism will allow the body to assimilate from the food or, when necessary, from herbs, all of the potassium phosphate it requires.

We must know and rule ourselves before we can properly utilize the organic cell salts. For they are mineralized expression of the twelve spiritual forces represented by the zodiac which will purify and refine us physically and set us free to express fully the Life Principles in conformity with our highest ideals.

Through the science of astrology we may learn wherein we fail to accomplish. Astrology is the finest method of self-analysis and self-perfection and is a method well within reach of all.

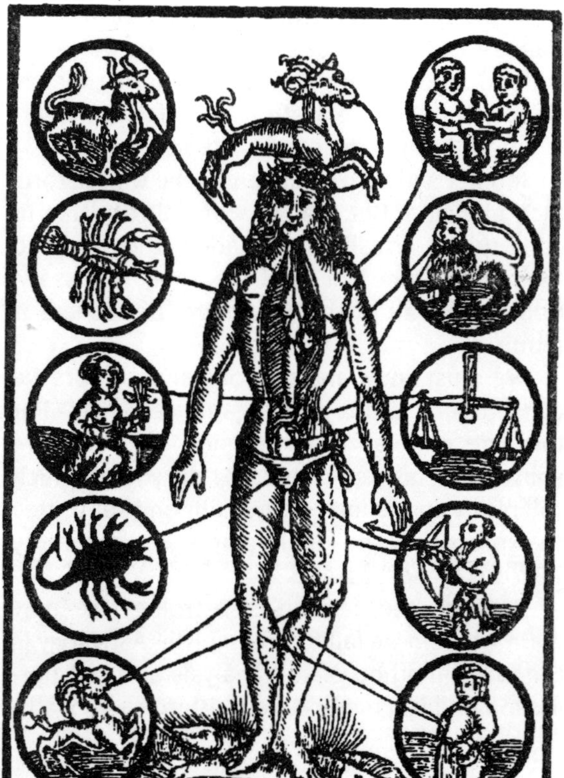

Health and the Sun Sign

We may liken the circle of the zodiac to a peal of 360 bells on one of which the note of our Sun is striking. If it is resonant, clear, and true, then we are living up to the highest we understand, in harmony with our environment.

If it is dull and discordant, then there is some weakness in the personal self and it has failed to respond to or recognize the solar harmony.

A knowledge of our solar strength will give us a consciousness of the realities of life and enable us to meet every situation and phase of life in calmness and gentleness.

The position of the Sun indicates the tone, the soul of the individual, divested of its phases and moods. It expresses itself in character, power, authority, dignity, self-reliance, and resolution according to the sign it was in at birth.

It represents our faith. It is the center of our being and it will show how the soul powers may be put forth and the capacity for soul growth during this life.

The soul, typified by the birth sign, seeking expression, draws upon the physical reservoirs of strength and uses up certain mineral salts in excess of others. But when there is mental attunement, these are quickly supplied through food, air, and water, and physical balance is maintained.

The greater the obstacles the soul has created, the greater the physical depletion and mental inharmony and consequent delay in recognizing the needed supplies to repair the waste and build broken down body cells.

When we are expressing the highest we understand and thus eliminating negative states, we are attracted towards those foods which will supply the necessary waste. But the greater the violation of soul-consciousness and consequent emotional turmoil, the greater the tendency to pander to a depraved taste in the eating of unwholesome food.

The body that is feeble and sickly will be lacking in muscular endurance; the body that is coarse and heavy will lose touch with humanity through lack of refinement; and the one with the over-strained nervous system will be incapable of success in any line of endeavor that requires self-control.

A great responsibility rests upon the homemaker, a home can be marred if inappropriate food is supplied. Excesses of animal food and coarse vegetables will lower the vibrations of the body and coarsen it, but foods which ripen in the Sun will help the body to attain the vibrations necessary for it to breathe in the higher forces of peace, harmony, and self-control.

Most people are familiar with the signs of the Zodiac and know something of the attributes of the different signs. But to go a step further, to know the chemical affinity of the different signs, is to solve the food problems of the family.

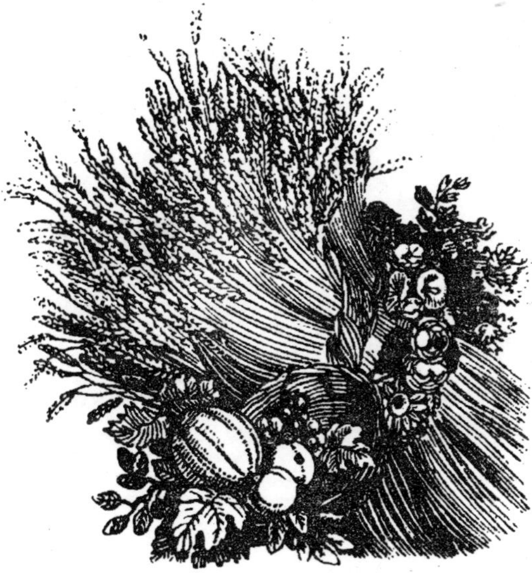

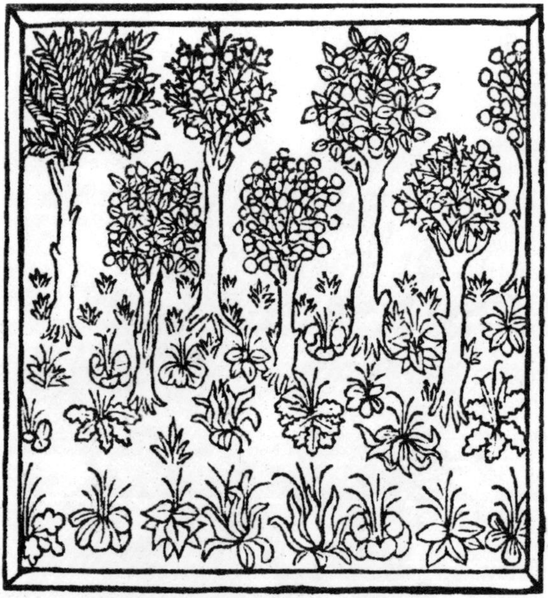

The Cell Salt of Aries

The Sun is passing through the sign Aries from about March 21 to April 20 each year and those born around sunrise during this period or when the sign Aries is on the Eastern horizon, which is two hours in every twenty-four, will tend to express the distinctly Aries nature. To a lesser extent, the Aries characteristics are displayed when the Moon is in the sign at the time of birth and when the Moon is passing through the sign in the progressed chart.

Aries endows its subjects with great activity of brain and body, with power to foresee and willingness to fight the battle of life. They always wish to be leaders and because of this as children they invariably associate with those younger than themselves.

They are intensely enthusiastic when their interest is aroused in a person or a cause. They are ambitious, self-willed, and impulsive. They have a passion for conquering and accomplishing more than the next man and in the more primitive types this expresses itself as extravagance in action, excess, chaos, and disruption. They appear to the outsider to be mere creatures of caprice.

Their desire for supremacy and leadersnip sometimes brings out the worst traits of jealousy, selfishness, and boasting but their passion for conquering eventually leads to self-conquering and then they become true leaders and comforters whether it be from the high official position or in the more lowly, comparatively obscure stations in life.

Potassium Phosphate is the cell salt of Aries and it takes its place in the scheme of human economy as the chemical base material expression and understanding. When either the Sun, Ascendant or Moon are in Aries there is great brain activity which calls for a steady replenishment of Potassium Phosphate. Unless the demand is met there is a break in the molecular chain of this brain and nerve builder and nervous disorders of all kinds result.

Potassium Phosphate in some mysterious way unites with albumen and transmutes it in to gray brain matter. It gives pliancy to the muscular tissue and is necessary for healthier liver action. A deficiency is soon manifested when there is excess mental action and insufficient rest, relaxation and repose. Instead of the earnest executive, determined brain worker we have the man who is irritable, unreliable, unfruitful, who sees slights where none are intended, whose judgment is warped and whose vision is out of focus.

Potassium Phosphate builds brain cells, strengthens nerve tissue, restores mental vigor provided that there is sufficient rest mentally and physically to help in the formation of new cells as the old ones decay. The Aries type perhaps more than any other needs to understand the meaning of relaxation and to practice it daily.

There is no difficulty in obtaining the daily supply of Potassium Phosphate as it is present in the commonest foods. Unlike some of the other cell-salts, it is not entirely spoiled through cooking the foods containing it, but in taking foods in an uncooked state it serves a double purpose in building brain and body cells and in neutralizing waste acids and it loses this latter power if the foods are cooked. The daily ration of the average individual contains much more Potassium Phosphate than the body requires in proportion to other cell salts but the body must reach a state of balance, equilibrium and repose that the required amount may be absorbed.

The foods containing most Potassium Phosphate are lettuce, cauliflower, olives, cucumbers, spinach, radishes, cabbage, potatoes, horseradish, onions, pumpkins, spinach, lima beans, lentils, walnuts, and apples.

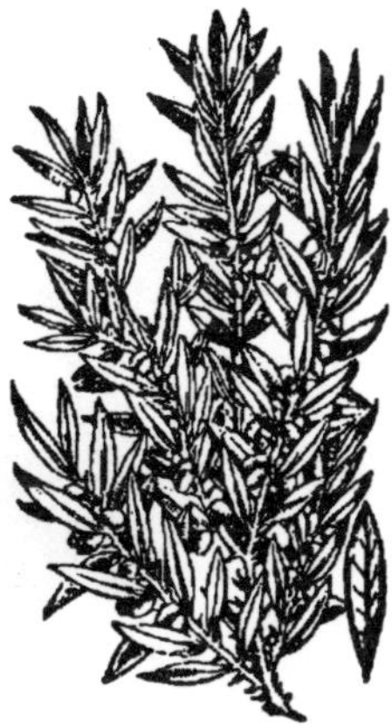

OLIVE

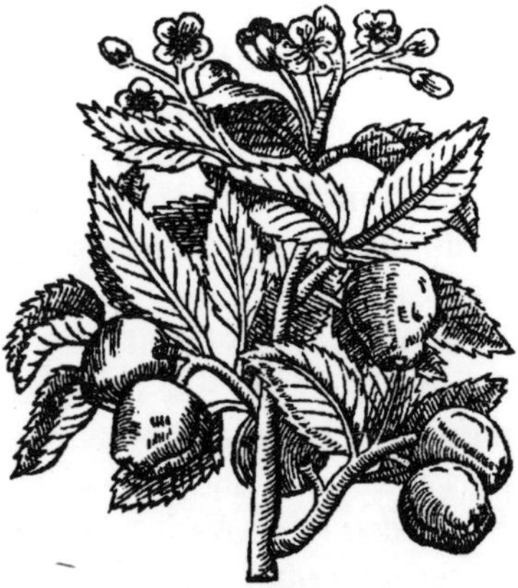

APPLE

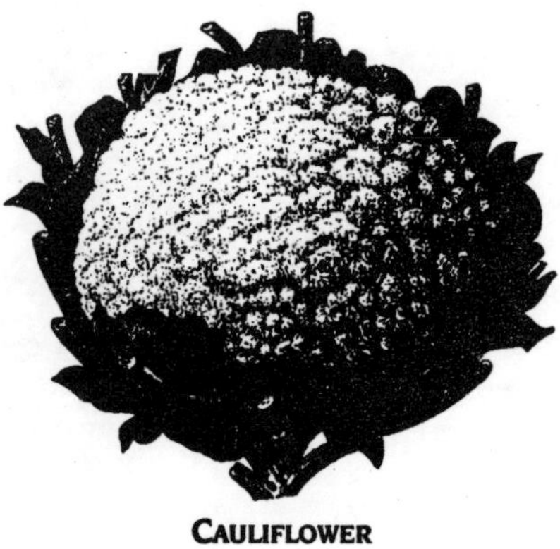

CAULIFLOWER

The Cell Salt of Taurus

The Sun is passing through the sign Taurus from April 19 to May 20 and those born about sunrise during this period or when the sign Taurus is on the Eastern Horizon, which is about two hours in every twenty-four, will tend to express the distinct Taurus nature. To a lesser extent the Taurus characteristics and the Taurus health condition will be noticed if the Moon is in that sign either in the birth chart or by progression.

Life seems to be full of changes and sorrows for the Taurus type, but these are brought about mainly through lack of poise and balance. The sign rules the lower brain and neck and represents the listening principle.

Creative energy, patience, and plodding perseverance are the chief characteristics, but too often passion rules and dominates and life's bitterest lessons are learned through misuse of their creative powers both on the mental and physical plane.

SULPHATE OF SODA is the cell salt of Taurus. Its mission is to control and regulate the supply of water in the body. It is present in the body in larger quantities in the liver, pancreas, and the liquids of the intercellular tissues.

Lack of this cell salt is first felt by heaviness at the base of the brain and an aching neck. This is followed by chill and fever. Usually the chilly stage is accompanied by night sweats, for sweating is nature's way of ridding the body of the excess water in the blood.

To rid the body of excess water due to a lack of Sulphate of Soda does not provide a remedy but merely a palliative; and unless the daily need of the cell salt is met, more serious health disturbances will result.

Those foods which keep the pores of the skin open and the body mobile are most in harmony with the sign Taurus and many of these also contain the necessary cell salt in the largest quantities. These are beet, spinach, horse radish, Swiss chard, cauliflower, cabbage, radish, cucumber, onions, and pumpkin.

The herbs most useful for condition are yarrow, burdock, and ground ivy, all of which are well-known and easily obtained. A drink made from an infusion of one of these will produce perspiration, rid the body of the superfluous water, and equalize the circulation besides supplying the necessary cell salt.

Mental and emotional balance and poise are very necessary for the Taurus type for health maintenance.

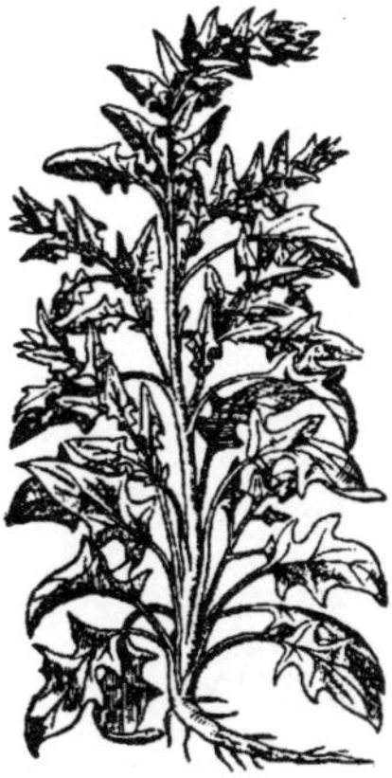

SPINACH

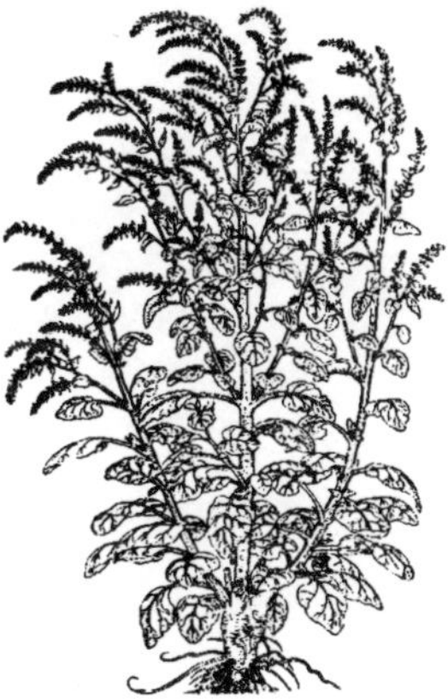

BEET

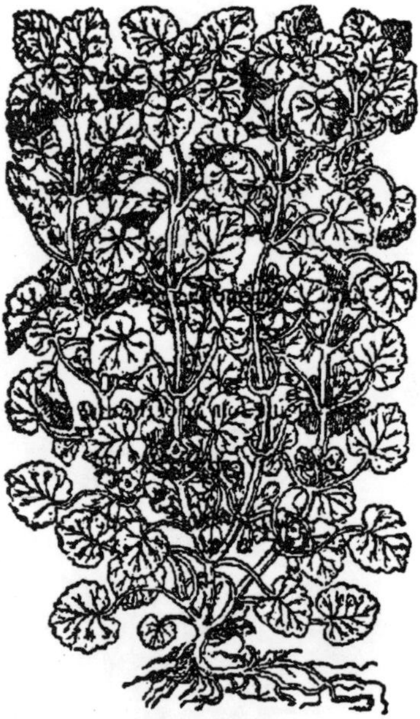

GROUND IVY

The Cell Salt of Gemini

The Sun is passing through the sign Gemini from May 22 to June 22 and those born during sunrise in this period or when the sign Gemini is on the Eastern Horizon, which is about two hours in every twenty-four, will tend to express the distinctly Gemini nature. To a lesser extent the Gemini characteristics and health condition will be noticed if the Moon is in that sign either in the birth chart or by progression.

Gemini represents thought, the instrument through which man may rule and conquer and attain his object, hence people ruled by Gemini should do their best work in mental and intellectual fields.

Gemini also rules the hands and arms and so we find Gemini natives efficient and happy in work which requires the combined use of hand and the head, such as painting, publishing, writing, printing, etc.

As they reach the higher mental states they are susceptible to the influence of inspirational currents and so make good orators. They have a passion for knowledge which ranges from self-knowledge to an interest in a neighbor's welfare and all that that implies; from mathematical studies to the study of Divine mathematics according to the sign and aspects of their ruler Mercury.

The Cell Salt of Gemini is **POTASSIUM CHLORIDE**. This salt builds and regulates the fibrin in the blood. A deficiency of Potassium Chloride results in a thickening of the fibrin and this must be thrown out by way of the glands and mucous membrane or it will form into little balls and block the circulatory system and death ensues.

The normal proportion of fibrin in the human blood is only 3 parts in 1,000, yet as small as this amount is, an increase to 5 or 6 parts in 1,000 shows itself in diseases such as pleurisy, pneumonia, diphtheria, etc., through an effort of Nature to throw out the excess fibrin.

The herbs most useful in this condition are meadowsweet, tansy, vervain, yarrow, as these contain large quantities of Potassium Chloride and appear to quickly dissolve in the thickening blood.

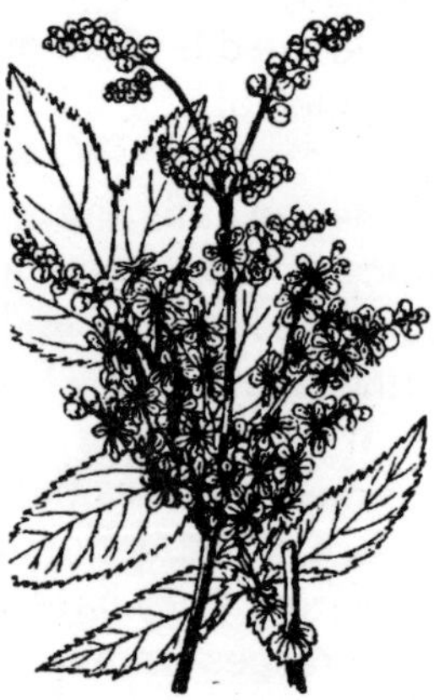

MEADOWSWEET

The foods most useful in this condition are asparagus, corn, green beans, beets, sprouts, carrots, cauliflower, spinach, tomatoes, sweet celery, oranges, peaches, pineapple, apricots, pears, and plums, some of these should form part of the menu of every day of the Gemini native, but the cell salt necessary will only be absorbed and assimilated by the body to the extent that mental activities are regulated, controlled, and directed.

The mission of Gemini is to elevate mankind through sympathetic understanding from the animal plane to that of the higher plane; to investigate those sciences that promote commerce; to contact the Astral Light first, through expressing the highest understanding, and then through a realization of this, putting it into practice in daily life.

To fall below the ideal in thought is to limit the practical expression of it and the body is consequently disrupted, for as thought and expression are repressed or turned upon self, so is the circulation of the blood slowed up resulting in the non-elimination of excess fibrin, the element of expression.

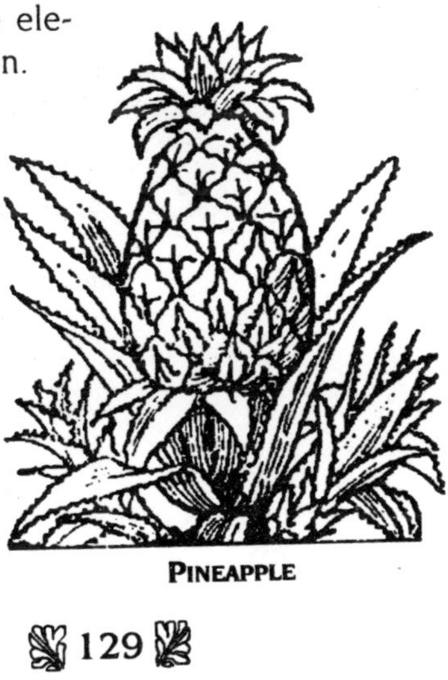

PINEAPPLE

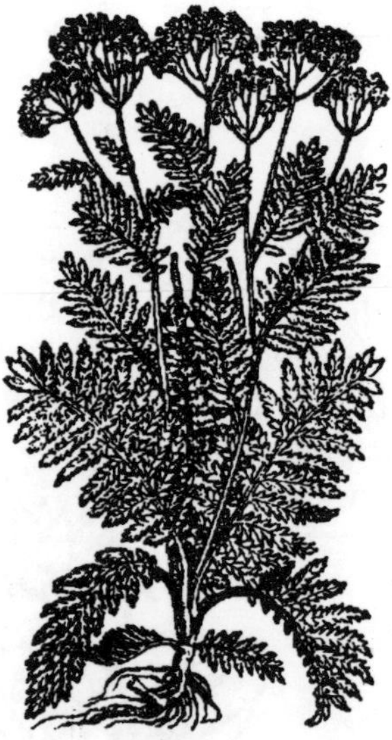

YARROW

The Cell Salt of Cancer

The Sun is passing through the sign Cancer from June 22 to July 22, and those born at sunrise during this period or when the sign Cancer is on the Eastern Horizon, which is about two hours in every twenty four, will tend to express the distinctly Cancer nature. To a lesser extent the Cancer characteristics and health condition will be noticed when the Moon is passing through that sign either in the birth chart or by progression. There is also noticed an adverse condition of the health and lowered vitality when there is a malefic in Cancer and an adverse aspect of the Moon.

Cancer governs the powers of inspiration and respiration. Personal experiences in the outer world and the perfecting of his attitude towards these is the food for man in his pilgrimage. Cancer is the sign of inflowing, but just what will flow in depends upon where the Moon, the ruler of Cancer, is positioned in the birth chart.

The Cancer type is timid, retiring, and passive. They may seem slothful, but they are incessant workers on the mental plane and when in a condition of health, mentally and physically, the spiritual and material forces are well balanced and they possess reflective power of a very high order.

They are great lovers of home and family and the desire for perfection in their belongings often causes a worrying habit until members of the family are driven away from them. The desire for recognition, which is very strong in this type, saps their nervous energy and they become a monument of selfishness or helplessness in the eyes of all with whom they come in contact.

Fluoride of Lime is the Cell Salt of Cancer, and in the tense, all wound up condition caused by reacting to impressions of that which he does not recognize as himself, the Cancer subject soon suffers from Fluoride of Lime depletion.

Fluoride of Lime combines with albumen and oil to preserve the elasticity of the fibre of the connective tissue in the body. There are traces of it in the enamel of the teeth and in the iris of the eye.

Lack of it causes relaxed conditions of tissue as in varicose veins, falling of the womb, decay of the teeth, curvature of the spine, and weakened eyesight.

Sometimes the lack is first apparent in the break of the magnetic or electric currents between the upper and lower brain poles and a mental condition bordering on insanity through groundless fears of various kinds is the result.

Fluoride of Lime is found in most animal and vegetable foods but in largest quantities in the yolk of eggs and in whole rye flour. The mental balance, however, must be partly restored

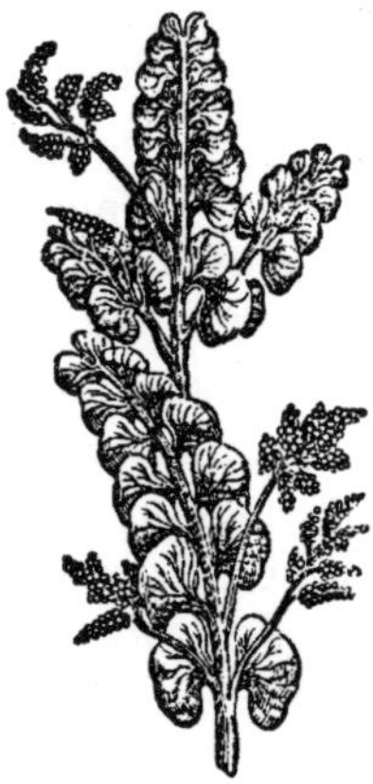

MOONWORT

before the body can assimilate it. If food were all in health restoration, then it would be a simple matter to choose that which contains the necessary cell salt in the largest proportion; but food nourishes only that which is taken when the body is in a relaxed, easy condition.

Apprehension, fear, dread, anger, worry, and jealousy all keep the body tense and cause psychic or mental tumors and create a bodily condition or breeding-ground for physical tumors and cancers.

The Cancer type and those with a malefic planet afflicted in Cancer are the greatest sufferers from tumorous and cancerous complaints.

Generous, peaceful thoughts build up the body and allow it to preserve its elasticity by extracting from the food sufficient Fluoride of Lime, but niggardly thoughts and violent emotions tear down, and the effects of these are first apparent in the person originating these thoughts. Ailments fall upon each with equal justice and impartiality.

Tired out, filled with indefinable fears, allowing feeling to steal the will, one fit of intense emotion will unbalance for life.

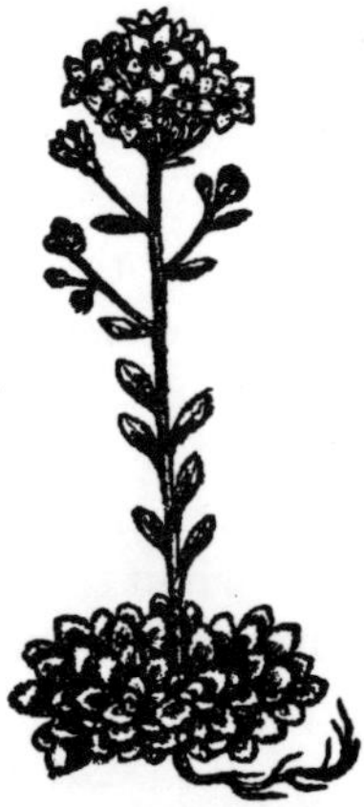

SAXIFRAGE

Deep down in the depths of our inner consciousness, far from the maddening problems of the personality, is the knowledge of all law.

Nervous energy acts in response to the mind and its vibrations are governed by the dominant mental impressions. Thorough relaxation is very necessary for the Cancer type. They may then more readily refuse thoughts manufactured by tension and with the freer circulation of nervous energy, raise their consciousness to those aspirational heights of which they dream in their more restful moments.

The most helpful foods for Cancer afflictions are milk, eggs, cabbage, lettuce, watercress, and pumpkin. The herbs are chickweed, saxifrage, willow, wintergreen, water violet, purslain, privet, and moonwort.

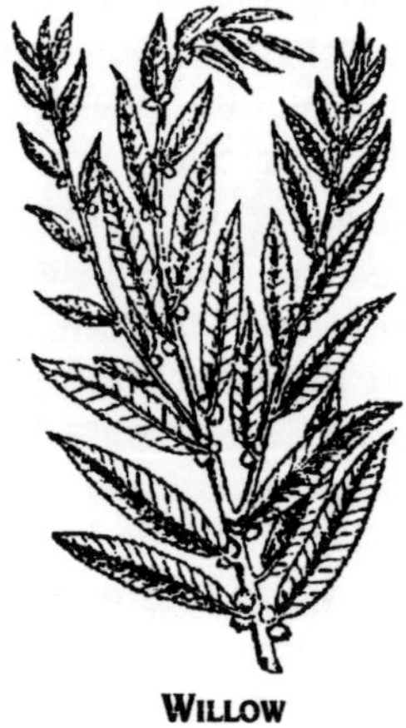

WILLOW

The Cell Salt of Leo

The Sun is passing through the sign Leo from July 23 to August 23, and those born at sunrise during this period or when Leo is in the Eastern Horizon, which is about two hours in every twenty-four, will tend to express the distinct Leo nature. To a lesser extent the Leo characteristics and health condition will be noticed when the Moon by progression is passing through Leo and by those having the Moon in the birth chart in the sign Leo.

Phosphate of Magnesia is the cell salt of the Leo type, and they consume more of that cell salt than any other. When we consider that all of the blood from all parts of the body goes through the heart and that Leo rules the heart, how necessary it is that a sufficient supply of the Leo cell salt should be consumed that the blood returning may be revivified.

The Leo type moves upon the sensitive and emotional planes and is fiery and intuitive, hasty and impulsive. Under the influence of emotional stress they will often act without thinking, and the more primitive types, when roused to the pitch of passionate fury, seem insane in their wild and erratic actions. Like the lion, an intense degree of excitement blinds them.

The more awakened of this type will follow impulsively some mental genius, particularly if they have the courage to depart from the beaten track or to proclaim some new truth or philosophy. The mental force within them is ever striving to reach some higher level, but they require the association of those dominated by one of the air signs.

Phosphate of Magnesia will restore their lost nervous force and muscular vigor. It gives the skeleton its firmness as well as helping to form the albumen in the blood. It vitalizes brain and nerves and it invigorates the excretory organs and helps to maintain the natural fluidity of the blood.

Foods containing Phosphate of Magnesia in the largest quantities are barley, whole wheat

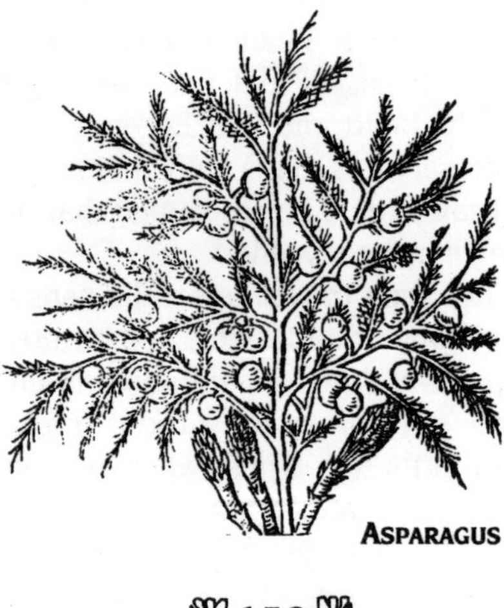

Asparagus

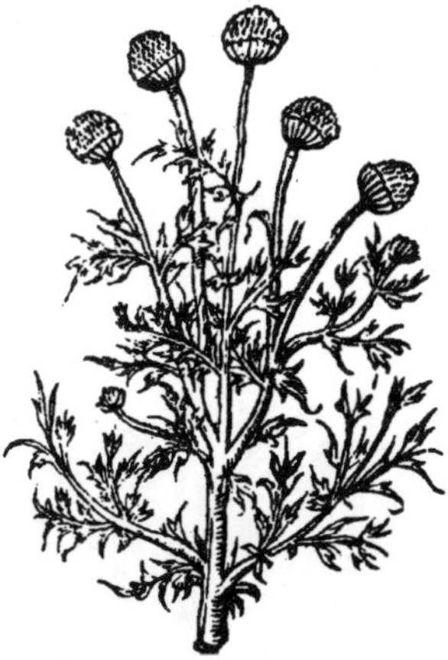

CHAMOMILE

bread, rye, almonds, lettuce, apples, figs, asparagus, eggs, cabbage, cucumber, coconut, walnuts, blueberries, and onions.

The herbs under the Leo sign are dill, fennel, comfrey, chamomile, St. John's wort, marigold, parsley, and garden mint.

Phosphate of Magnesia in its commercial form is harmful and cannot be assimilated by the body but a sufficient quantity can be obtained from the foods mentioned, provided there is not excessive meat eating. The Leo type, possibly more than any other, should abstain from all stimulating foods and beverages, as these tend to keep them on that plane wherein they are ruled by the senses. There they develop craft and cunning which kills intelligence and prevents the proper exercise of the intuitional faculties.

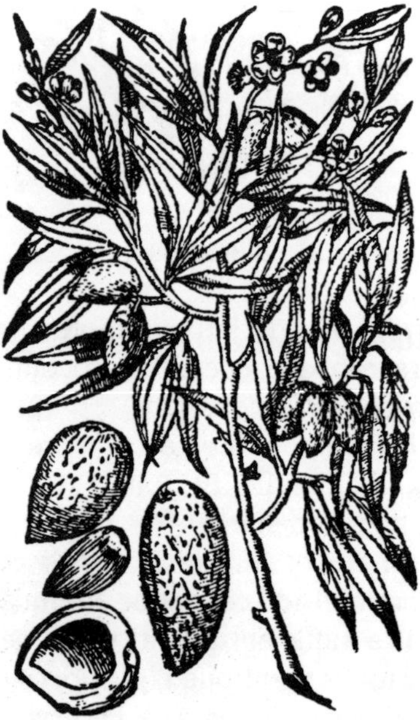

ALMOND

The Cell Salt of Virgo

The Sun is passing through Virgo from August 23 to September 22 and those born at sunrise during this period or when Virgo is on the Eastern horizon, which is about two hours in every twenty-four, will tend to express the distinctly Virgo nature.

To a lesser extent the Virgo characteristics and health condition are noticed when the Moon, by progression, is passing through Virgo and by those having the Moon in the sign Virgo in their birth chart.

As with the other signs, there are three very distinct Virgo types. The more primitive types show a great deal of selfishness and destructive criticism. A more advanced type tends to turn their criticism upon themselves and through introspective habits become too mentally sensitive. A third type is calm, contented, practical, and reflective—a repository of knowledge and an efficient employee.

Generally speaking, it is a sign keenly alive to its own interests but all born under it tend to echo their environment. The Virgos are the workers, the Marthas who are interested in many things, but who criticize the compassionate

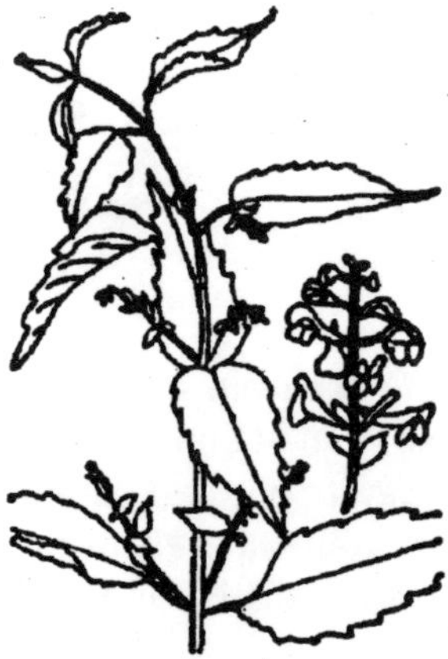

Skullcap

Mary, until, through experience, mother love is born in them, as they recognize the Divinity of true compassion.

The Virgo is not usually successful in business for himself, owning either to his want of confidence or lack of judgment, but through discernment, industry, and perseverance in the employ of others, he often reaches a position of comparative affluence.

The Cell Salt of Virgo is **Potassium Sulphate**. This works in the albumenoids, and in the oil in the human economy. Deficiency of Potassium Sulphate results in the thickening of the oil and the consequent clogging of the pores of the skin. Lack of it is shown in the liver when it fails to set free sufficient bile. In the scalp deficiency is shown by falling hair, scurf, dandruff, etc.

When the pores of the skin are partially closed through the thickening of the oil, body impurities, which should leave in the perspiration, are thrown back on the internal organs and coughs, colds, nasal catarrh, pleurisy, pneumonia, etc., result as the body tries to free itself by other means.

The Virgo weakness of destructive criticism reacts on the body rendering it unable to assimilate its cell salt. The sixth house principle is "We cannot hurt another except through ourselves and the seeds of self-destruction are already sown in he who wilfully and maliciously detracts from the merits of another."

The Hindu Astrologers regarded Virgo as the sign of enemies. It is undoubtedly a sign of struggle, but struggle leading to love—that tender sympathy which shines on all alike and finally obtains liberty through an understanding of what constitutes true freedom for others.

Virgo has been typified as a woman clothed with the Sun (Individuality) but having the Moon (Personality) at her feet.

The foods containing the Virgo cell salt in the largest proportion are endive, chicory, carrot, whole wheat, oats, rye and most salad vegetables. The best known herbs are valerian, skullcap, and privet.

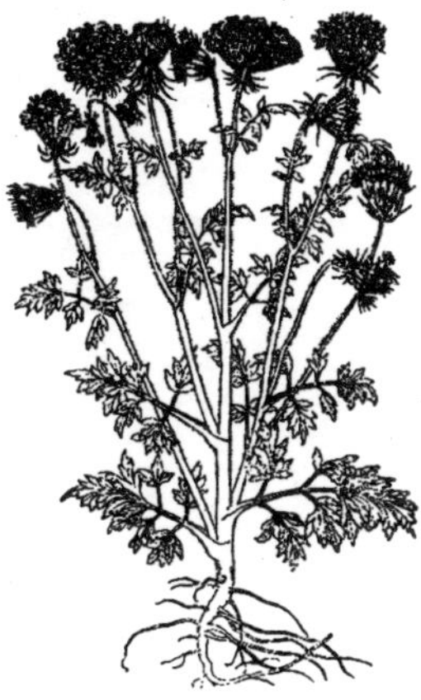

CARROT

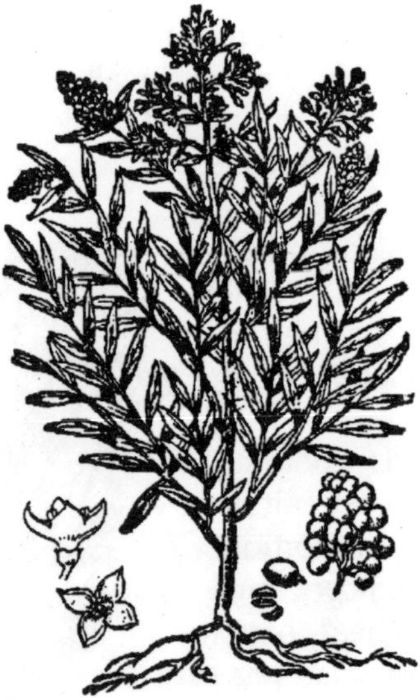

PRIVET

The Cell Salt of Libra

The Sun is passing through the sign Libra from September 23 to October 23 and those born at sunrise during this period or when Libra is on the eastern horizon, which is nearly two hours in every twenty-four, will tend to express the distinctly Libra characteristics and health condition.

To a lesser extent, these are noticed if the Moon in the birth chart is in Libra and when the Moon by progression is passing through the sign.

People born during the morning hours when the Sun is in Libra are keenly perceptive. They sense affection or aversion in others but, even in spite of very strong aversions, they are broad-minded and readily excuse the seeming weaknesses in others.

They possess originality and the capacity for leadership and their kindly encouragement inspires others, providing they are not too patronizing. They know how to find the easiest methods of working.

They will give name, fame, or fortune for a cause in which they are interested, yet they usually move in very exclusive circles.

The Librans are successful in business because, as a rule, they are broad-minded and optimistic and above petty fault-finding habits and criticism. They possess an abundance of ready-made tact, social charm and all-round ability. They hate injustice and unfairness and their gently persuasive ways make them good teachers of music and art.

The cell salt of Libra is **Sodium Phosphate** and, just as the sign Libra is represented as the Balance, so the work of its cell salt is to maintain the balance between acids and alkalis.

Worry through lack of appreciation, followed by fear, pessimism, and domestic inharmony, increases the acid condition of the body and makes a greater demand on the Sodium Phosphate. Sodium Phosphate is one of the laundrymen of the body, helping it to expel carbonic acid through the lungs and other carbonaceous waste through the skin and bladder.

If humans were mere mechanisms responding to food only, giving them doses of Sodium Phosphate would be like converting the world from selfishness to Altruism and Love, for the perfect balance between the acids and the fluids of the nerves, stomach, liver, and brain would mean perfect harmony; but humans are not mere mechanisms and the selfish temptation towards competition, business rivalry, envy, strife, and jealousy all disturb that perfect balance and harmony and there wages an eternal conflict be-tween spirit and matter.

To avoid denatured foods and have a plentiful supply of those foods rich in Sodium Phosphate will tend towards physical harmony in revitalizing the kidneys and bladder, for these are the physical seats of domestic inharmony. Striving for physical health will sometimes bring about mental readjustment.

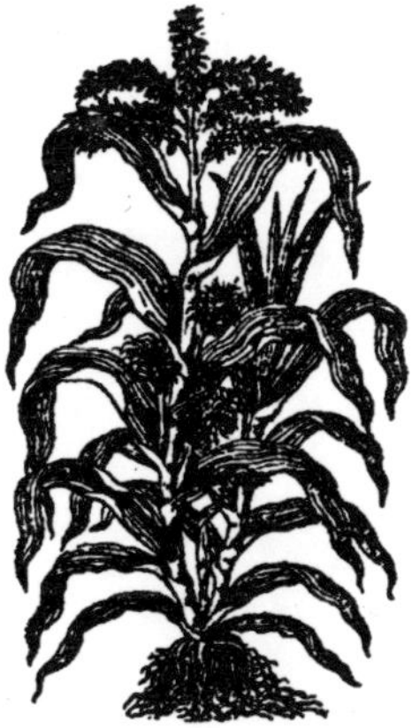

Corn

The foods containing the Libra cell salt in the largest quantities are celery, carrots, spinach, asparagus, beets, peas, yellow corn, strawberries, apples, figs, blueberries, raisins, almonds, fresh coconut, oatmeal, wheat, and unpolished rice. The herbs of Libra are watercress, violet, balm, and thyme.

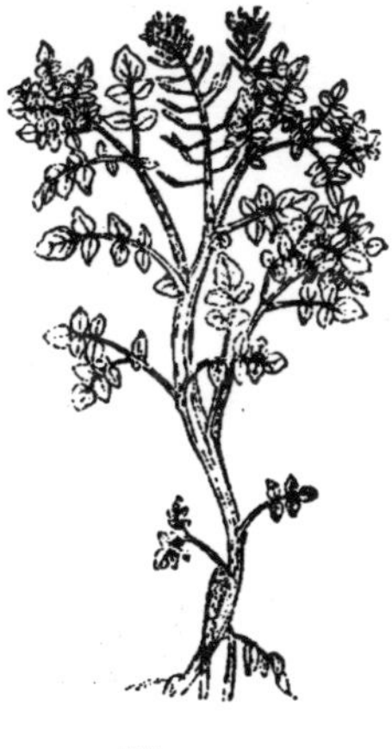

Watercress

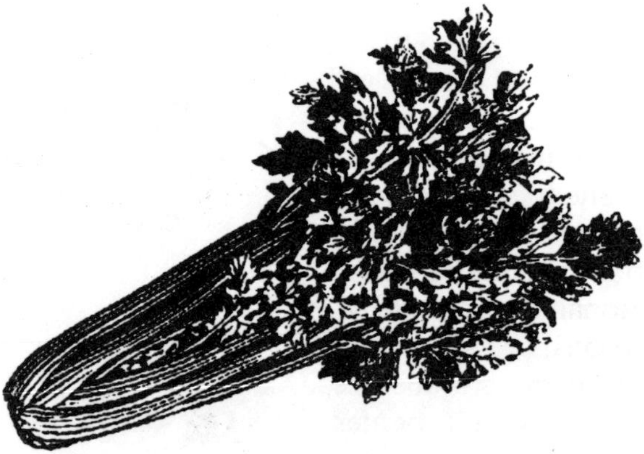

CELERY

The Cell Salt of Scorpio

The Sun is passing through the sign Scorpio from October 23 to November 22 and those born at sunrise during this period or when Scorpio is on the Eastern Horizon, which is nearly two hours in every twenty-four, will tend to express the distinctly Scorpio characteristics and health condition. To a lesser extent these are noticed if the Moon in the birth chart is in Scorpio or when the Moon by progression is passing through the sign.

People born under the Scorpio sign are subject to great extremes in life and there is no other sign which furnishes us with such extremes in character. In the lower types we can see the reason for the name "Scorpio" for, like their prototype, their bite is venomous and in their senseless anger their poisonous sting directed against others in impotent rage returns to themselves, stinging them into sickness or even death, unless their better nature should assert itself.

Scorpio is the emblem of generation and life and in this sign more than in any other there is a battle with the subtle force of sex attraction, which may be degraded by lust or, through self-control, transmuted so their emotional depths may find conscious expression in an awakened intuition.

The true Scorpion of the higher type has an inexhaustible resource of ideas and suggestions. His evolutionary mind is always busy with some new project. He has keen perceptive faculties, fine intuitional, powers and a very positive will.

Many successful physicians are born under the sign Scorpio but their success lies mainly in the abundant magnetic life force, which they possess and sympathetically transmit to their patients.

The possibilities of the Scorpio people are boundless after they have passed through the trials and tribulations necessary to subdue personalities and to teach caution, or when they have been toned by education and the environment necessary for their development.

Sulphate of Lime is the Scorpio cell salt. A break in the molecular chain of this cell salt disturbs the astral fluids and the grey matter of the brain and this break may be the result of wrong diet, but it more often occurs through over-work and dissipation and instead of the resourcefulness which is inherent in this type we have excess of pride, vanity, and a selfish disregard for the rights of others.

Sulphate of Lime works in the fibrine and helps to build epithelial tissue. It maintains the natural resisting power of the body through its cleansing and anti-septic powers, throwing impurities to the surface of the body so decay and injury to adjoining tissue may be prevented.

Deficiency of Sulphate of Lime results in thickening of the fibrine and the first warning of this condition may be either catarrh or a few pimples. Change of diet and mental readjustment and harmony will be all that is necessary at this stage, but deficiency of Sulphate of Lime may so weaken the resisting power of the body that more serious disorders such as pleurisy, pneumonia, and diphtheria may develop.

Sulphate of Lime can only be absorbed by the body and used in tissue-building in the form in which it is found in plant life, commercial Sulphate of Lime being too coarse to be absorbed; and the body will only absorb the necessary amount from the food to the extent that the spiritual essence of Sulphate of Lime, the purification of the senses, is expressed in the life for the Cell Salts of the Zodiac are the material expressions of their spiritual counterparts and, just as in mental and spiritual inharmony distort our understanding of unity and oneness, to that extent they render the body incapable of transmuting the physical expressions of divine principles into bodily health.

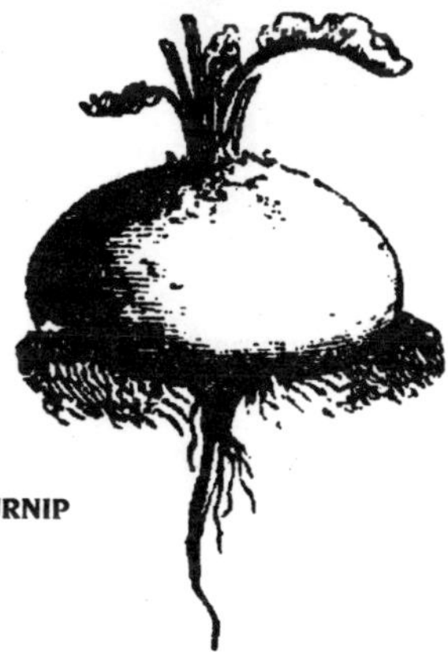

TURNIP

The foods containing Sulphate of Lime in larger quantities are onions, asparagus, kale, garlic, mustard, cress, turnips, figs, cauliflower, radishes, leeks, prunes, black cherries, gooseberries, blueberries, and coconut. The herbs containing the Scorpio cell salt are nettles, horehound, butterbur, and wormwood.

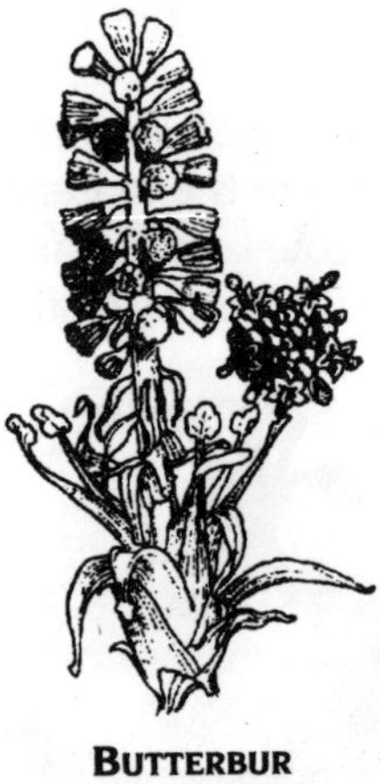

Butterbur

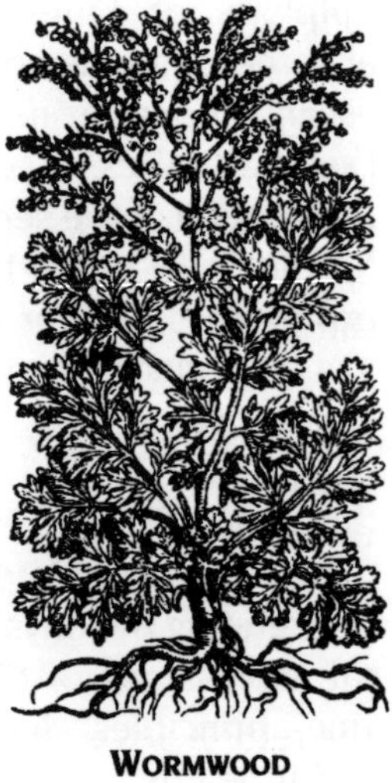

Wormwood

The Cell Salts of Sagittarius

The Sun is passing through the sign Sagittarius from November 22 to December 21 and those born at sunrise during this period or when Sagittarius is on the Eastern Horizon which is about one and a half hours during every twenty-four, will tend to express the distinctly Sagittarius characteristics and health conditions.

To a lesser extent these are noticed if the Moon is in Sagittarius in the birth chart and when the Moon is progressing through the sign.

The Sagittarian works out his salvation through a dualistic career. Seldom do we find him with only one occupation, for no sooner is he launched in one line of work than he commences another, if only as a hobby—but he is thorough in whatever he undertakes to do.

His symbol is the archer, shooting with a straight and steady aim, and while he reaches his mark, he seems able to protect himself from the return blow for the time being.

His ready tongue and sarcastic wit often cruelly hurt his less clever associates although he seems quite unconscious of this, but if it is made known to him he quickly does all he can to make amends.

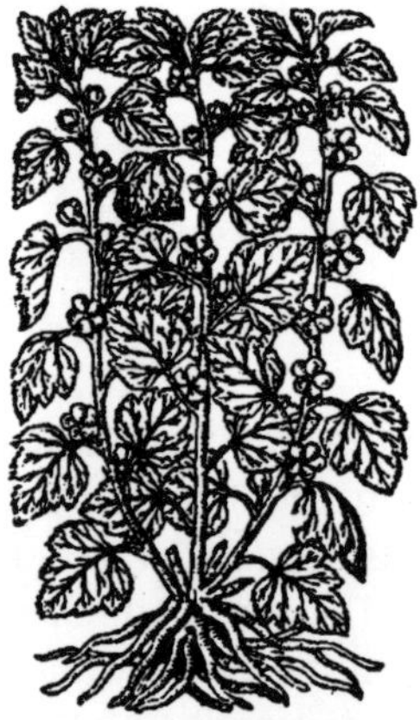

Marshmallow

Sagittarians will always take a sporting chance and if they follow their own intuitions, are rarely led astray, but in primitive and undeveloped types we find recklessness, rebelliousness, extravagance, carelessness, and indifference. Sagittarians are impatient where they do not comprehend and so are narrowminded.

The Sagittarian desires to do as the world does, and so is genial, sympathetic, courteous, and neutral, waiting to be led by a stronger force yet seeming to be a sound reasoner and logician externally.

The more highly evolved the type, the more keen the intuitive faculty. They seem to see through and demolish what others would find impenetrable barriers. They are equal to any emergency and inspire others with confidence in times of crisis.

They are clairvoyant, prophetic and inspired spiritual advisers, philanthropic, and compassionate but very just.

The cell salt of Sagittarius is **Silica** or common quartz. A deficiency of this is manifested in lack of luster in the hair, weak nails, and poor skin. Internally Silica is found in the covering of the bones and nerves and also in the bones.

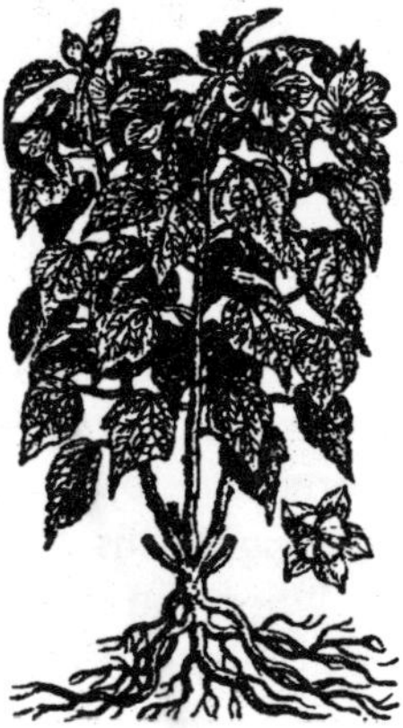
WATERMALLOW

Its office is to force to the surface all disintegrating foreign matter as pits, boils, pimples, etc., and heal and repair the surface. Healthy muscular tissue contains about two per cent of Silica and the pancreas contains no less than 12 per cent. A sufficiency of Silica helps to keep the body warm for it is a good insulator.

The skin of fruits and vegetables and the outer coats of cereals all contain Silica but most of this is thrown away in the preparation of food for human consumption.

Silica gives power of resistance to the stalks of grain and it is the material expression of the spiritual essence of resistance in mankind.

If Sagittarians have no higher aim in life than transitory pleasures, diversion, the desire for the good opinion of the crowd, intolerance of all that is foreign to their limited vision and prejudice if the Jupiterian qualities possessed are used selfishly to gain material success, their intuition becomes a source of evil since they can no longer contact the things of the spirit, and without these, intuition and perception avail nothing, seeming to give lavishly, only to take away all that is worth while.

True resistance, the spiritual essence of Silica, is manifested only as we have the courage to face every issue, to have faith in all that commends itself to both intuition and reason and to act upon it, neither seeking praise nor fearing censure.

The only form in which Silica can be used by the body is that found in plant life. It is contained in the edible skins of all fruits and vegetables as well as in figs, prunes, and strawberries.

It is found in most the pot-herbs which are commonly used as seasoning as well as in agrimony, feverfew, and the mallows, which are typical Sagittarius plants.

When the pancreas cannot assimilate sufficient Silica for its healthy activity, when morbid humors affect the bones and when the hair loses its gloss and the nails are weak and brittle, it may not be through lack of sufficient Silica in diet, but lack of power to raise that Silica to its highest potency that the body may use it. The plants absorb the Silica from the soil and thus gather the power to resist the winds that would destroy them.

We must gather the spiritual essence of Silica—resistance—grown of a faith which lives beyond all forms of faith, which will give our digestive system the power to extract and volatilize all of the Silica necessary from the food we eat.

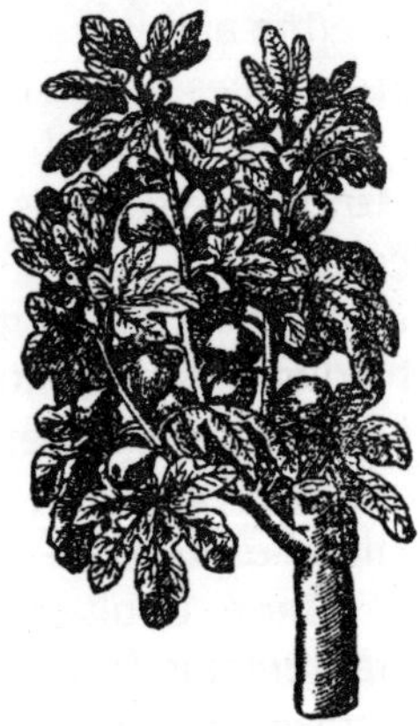

FIG

The Cell Salt of Capricorn

The Sun is passing through Capricorn from December 22 to January 21 and those born at sunrise during this period or when Capricorn is on the Eastern Horizon, which is nearly two hours in every twenty-four, will tend to express the distinctly Capricorn characteristics and health conditions.

To a lesser extent these will be manifest when the Moon in the birth chart is in Capricorn and also when the Moon, by progression, is passing through the sign.

The children of Capricorn and those with the sign Capricorn rising at the time of their birth are the greatest sufferers from rickets in infancy due to the lack of **CALCIUM PHOSPHATE** or **PHOSPHATE OF LIME** in their diet. The cell salt which is the chemical affinity of each sign must be daily replenished if health is to be maintained, and the mother of the Capricorn baby during nursing must see that her food is rich in the mineral salt that her child's body needs.

Then after being weaned, the Capricorn requires a plentiful supply of rich cow's milk, strawberry or blueberry juice in drinking water, or the liquid in which black figs have been boiled, to prevent rickets. Lime water, which is usually prescribed for rickets, is useless since the body cannot assimilate inorganic substances.

Calcium Phosphate carries albumen from the food to the bones and uses it to reconstruct and build new bone material, but if there is not enough Calcium Phosphate, the excess albumen leaves the body by way of the kidneys, resulting in disorders known as Bright's disease, stone and gravel, or it may find its way to the surface of the skin and manifest as boils and pimples. It may remain in the lungs, causing consumption, center in the nasal passages, causing catarrh, or lodge in the ear, causing deafness.

Deficiency of Phosphate of Lime causes irritation of the nerve terminations of the mucous membranes of the stomach and results in acids being formed from undigested foods which find their way to the joints, causing pain known as rheumatism.

The foods which contain the largest amount of Phosphate of Lime are strawberries, plums, blueberries, figs, spinach, asparagus, lettuce, cucumbers, almonds, coconut, lentils, brown beans, whole wheat, rye, barley, sea fish, and cow's milk.

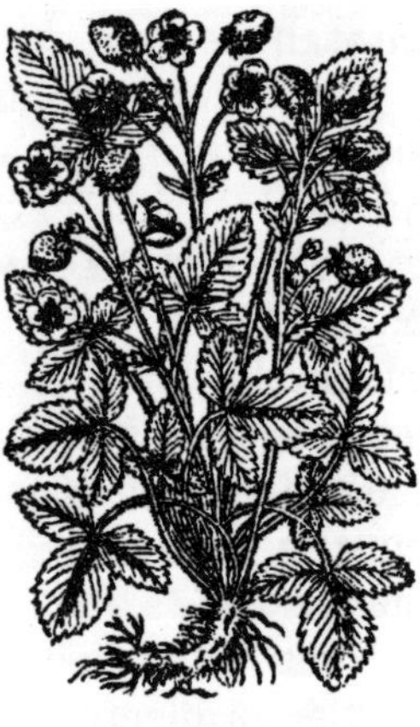

STRAWBERRY

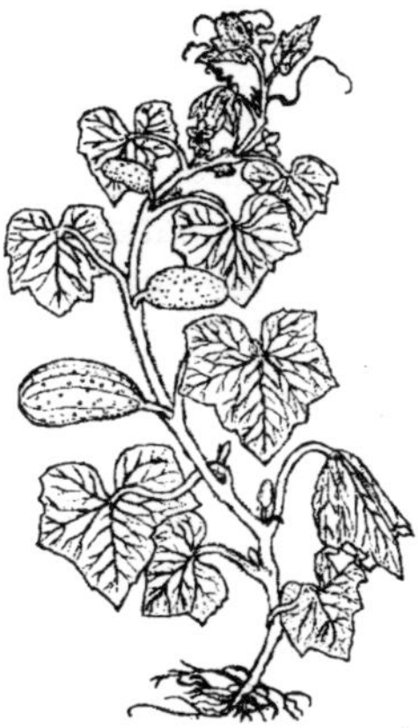

CUCUMBER

A knowledge of the birth charts with the progressed position of the Moon is a great help in understanding the physical disturbances of different members of the family, and a knowledge of the herbs ruled by the different signs is also essential.

As the Moon passes through the sign Capricorn by progression, even though it may be neither the sun nor ascending sign, physical disturbances of the nature of Capricorn will often be seen, thereby proving that the body can use up more Phosphate of Lime at that time than it is receiving.

In one instance which came under our notice, a large crop of warts appeared on the hands of a child as the Moon was passing through the first decanate of Capricorn. These were relieved by the juice of the knotweed, a Capricorn plant. Another child developed cramps and a troublesome cough. Mullein tea was given and the trouble disappeared. Earache, another Capricorn complaint, is quickly relieved by the juice of knotweed and stone in the kidneys is dissolved and passes easily away by a tea made from almost any Capricorn plant.

A balanced ration, in which the foods mentioned above have a prominent place, will prevent the diseases mentioned, but the herbs, which are merely foods in a more concentrated form, are often necessary in acute stages when a change of diet would be too slow in operation and entail unnecessary suffering.

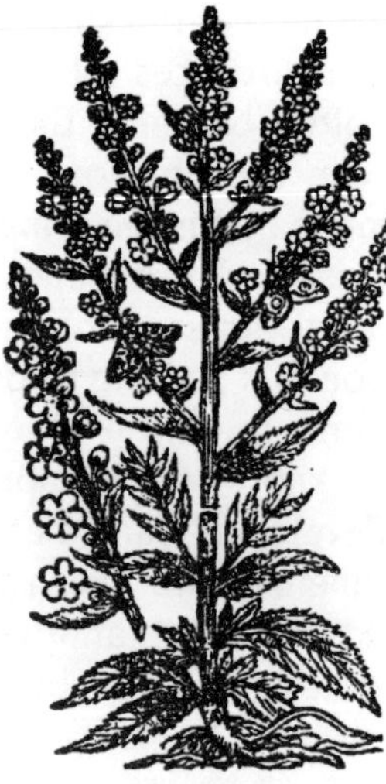

MULLEIN

The Cell Salt of Aquarius

The Sun is passing through Aquarius from January 20 to February 19 each year and people born at Sunrise during this period or when Aquarius is passing over the Eastern Horizon, which is nearly two hours in every twenty-four, will tend to express the distinctly Aquarius characteristics and health condition.

To a lesser extent this will be noticed if the Moon is in Aquarius in the birth chart and when the Moon, by progression, is passing through the sign.

Each sign has thirty degrees and those born while the Sun is in either of the first 10 degrees are remarkable for their intuitive brain and wonderful memory. The next 10 degrees of those born from February 1st to 10th, endow subjects with part of the nature of the knowledge absorbing intellect of the restless Gemini, while those born during the period from February 10th to 19th develop along musical and artistic lines and these do not usually exhibit the independent spirit of those during the earlier period and are too apt to rely on others.

The Aquarians usually follow unusual occupations or give an original turn to their work. They are capable of conducting original investigations, are interested the latest scientific discoveries, and generally speaking, have a mental attitude far in advance of their time.

Ruled by Uranus, that impulsive, uncertain, nervous, restless wanderer of the skies, they are eccentric, original, unconventional, loving mental freedom and independence, and are impatient of all control. There are no dull periods in the lives of those who have Uranus, the ruling planet of Aquarius, prominently placed in their birth charts for these are the makers of history.

Sodium Chloride is the cell salt of the Aquarian and the common name for Sodium Chloride is salt—table salt—but table salt is not a food but a preservative and is useful, if at all, in creating thirst. This it does by acting upon the mucous membrane of the digestive tract and absorbs the water therefrom and the demand is made for more water to supply the deficiency.

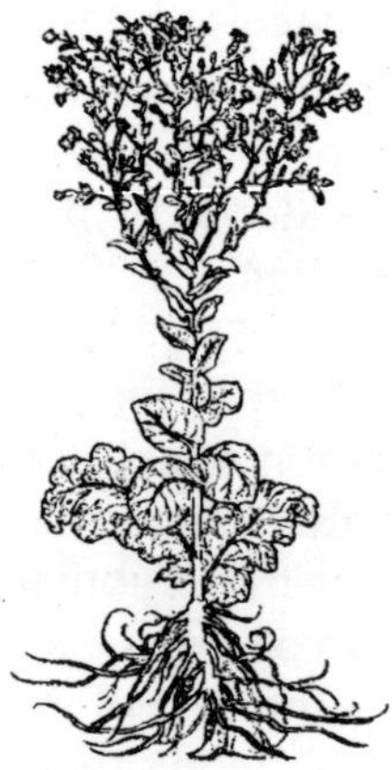

Lettuce

Common salt will attract towards it the moisture in a room, which is easily proven by leaving a quantity of it in a damp kitchen. Sodium Chloride in the body attracts and carries and dis-

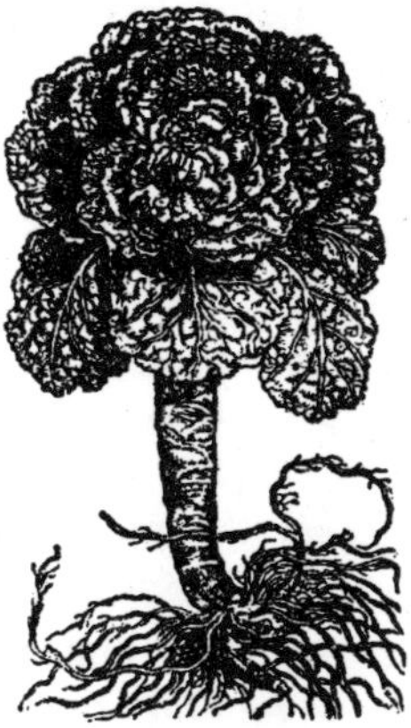

CABBAGE

tributes the water in the human organism.

When water is not properly distributed in the body, the delicate fibres that form a network through every inch of human anatomy feel and express vibrations of in-harmony.

The influence of the Sun in Aquarius or the Moon by progression through that sign tends to the elimination of salt and on the first symptom of disease, the first call is for some food that is rich in sodium chloride.

The human body is about 70 per cent water so a cell salt's whole mission is to unite with and make water useful, just as the salty liquid is necessary in the proper working of the electric battery, must necessarily be supplied and absorbed in large proportion.

When there is a deficiency of sodium chloride the continuity of the molecular chain of water is broken and illusions, sometimes amounting to insanity will often result. Common salt is too coarse to be absorbed by the blood and the only form of sodium chloride that the body can use is that in plant form which has been absorbed from the soil.

The Aquarians, through their mental action, consume more of this cell salt which controls the moisture in the body than any other type.

The deficiency can only be supplied by a change of diet or by strengthening the digestive organs so that they can extract from it the food in which it has been stored direct from the soil.

The foods containing the largest amount of sodium chlorate are strawberries, apples, figs, spinach, cabbage, radish, asparagus, carrots, cucumber, lettuce, chestnuts, coconuts and lentils.

Sometimes it happens that a more concentrated food is required through the emergency of the case, then it is that we may safely resort to herbs, provided we choose the herbs in sympathy with the rising sign. The herbs in sympathy with Uranus are: Southernwood, valerian, comfrey root and leaves, and the bayberry. These assist by supplying the necessary salt in more concentrated form and in giving tone to the digestive system that it may extract all that is necessary from the food eaten, since it is not what we eat but what is assimilated that builds and strengthens the body.

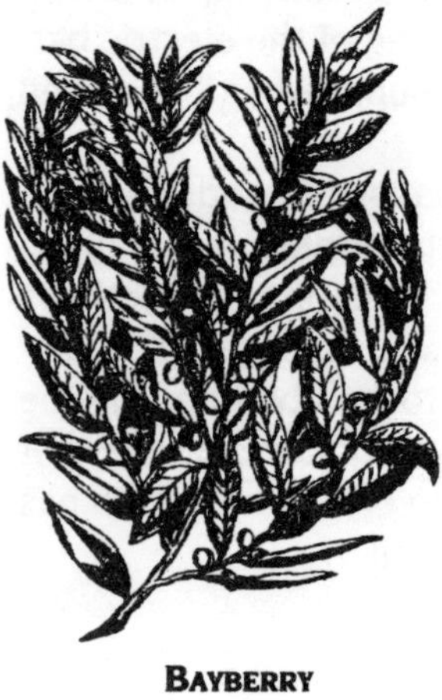

Bayberry

The Cell Salt of Pisces

The Sun is passing through Pisces from February 20 to March 24 and those born at sunrise during this period or when the sign Pisces is on the Eastern Horizon will tend to express the distinctly Pisces characteristics and health condition.

To a lesser extent this will be noticed when the Moon is in Pisces in the birth chart, and when it is passing through Pisces in the progressed chart.

Those born when the Sun, Moon, or Ascendant are in Pisces will tend to use up a great deal of the cell salt **Phosphate of Iron**, and if it is not replenished daily, chronic ill-health is the result.

A characteristic of those born while one of the sensitive points above mentioned is in Pisces, is a predisposition to over-anxiety, worry, indulging in gloomy forebodings, and they have many experiences in life that are far from pleasant.

Their sympathies are easily awakened for all who suffer and they are very receptive to the moods of those in their environment. This receptivity is too often a stumbling block, increasing their anxiety but limiting their power to help until, through command of their lower emotional nature, they can control the situation, and through equilibrium, themselves.

Their internal aspirations are very high. They are very ambitious and they have power to occupy a prominent position through merit and adaptability to environment. Until they can free themselves from anxiety, restlessness, and the desire for appreciation which sometimes expresses itself in selfishness, jealousy, and pride, they will be subject to the physical weakness characteristic of the sign.

Lack of Phosphate of Iron, the cell salt of Pisces, results in an inflammatory condition that leads to coughs, colds, chills, fevers, pneumonia and various glandular ulcerations. Iron is the carrier of oxygen and without sufficient Iron, health is impossible, but the only iron that can be used by the body is that in organic molecules and the body cannot use these unless there is also a desire to understand the cause of the health disturbance and use the remedy which lies within themselves, mental control.

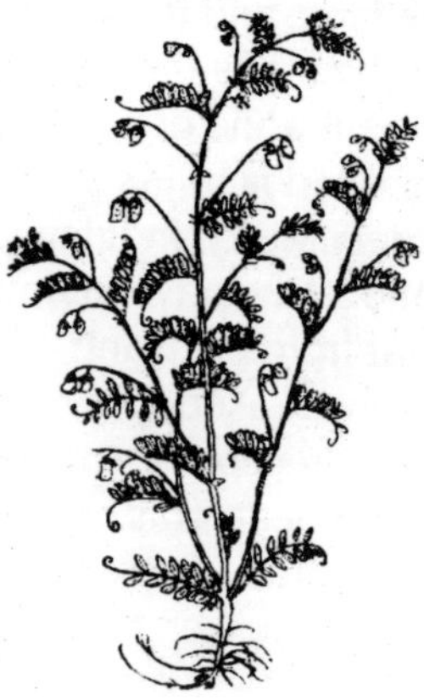

Lentils

Iron's affinity for oxygen is well known. Leave Iron exposed to the air for a time and it attracts sufficient oxygen out of the air to form Iron Oxide, Fe_3O_4,

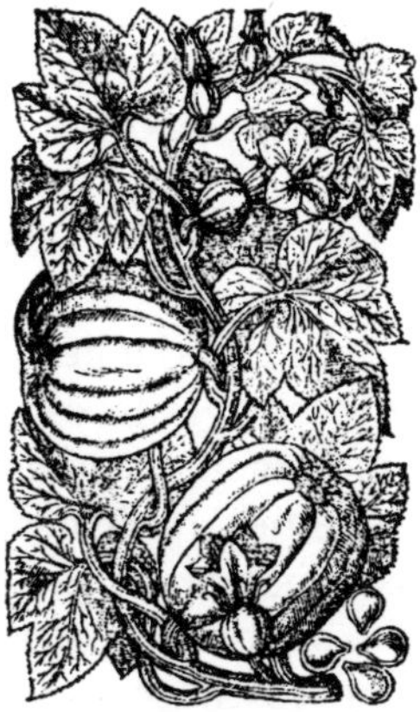

PUMPKIN

generally known as iron rust. In similar manner, iron attracts the oxygen taken in in the form of food and air and distributes it to strengthen the blood vessels and arteries.

When these is a lack of Iron, blood is drawn from the surface of the skin to carry on important work in more vital centers of the body, and the complexion is pale and anemic looking and the pores of the skin are less active. The poisons which should leave the body by the skin accumulate as mucous membrane and show their presence by means of colds, catarrh, pleurisy, etc. The Turkish bath and other sweating processes may free the skin temporarily and remove much of the poisonous waste, but unless the cause is removed—deficiency of Phosphate of Iron—the sweat bath may result in more harm than good.

Absence of iron may finally lead to dropsy, glandular diseases, tonsillitis, inflammation of the bladder, diphtheria, relaxed muscles, bedwetting in children, granulated eyelids, inflammatory neuralgia, mumps, croup, etc.

In all fevers there is a lack of Phosphate of Iron. The blood cannot get a sufficient supply of oxygen unless the Iron is also there and so the circulatory system is speeded up and a feverish condition is the result.

Foods that are eaten to act as a tonic in conditions mentioned above should not be cooked, as cooking sets free the Iron, changes it to tincture of Iron, and it is thrown away by most cooks in the water used for boiling.

Phosphorus and iron are to be found together in some foods, such as spinach, lentils, cabbage, onions, barley. Iron is present in large quantities in lettuce, strawberries, radishes, horseradish and phosphorus in pumpkins, lima beans, cucumbers, almonds, walnuts, apples and potato skins in addition to those mentioned above.

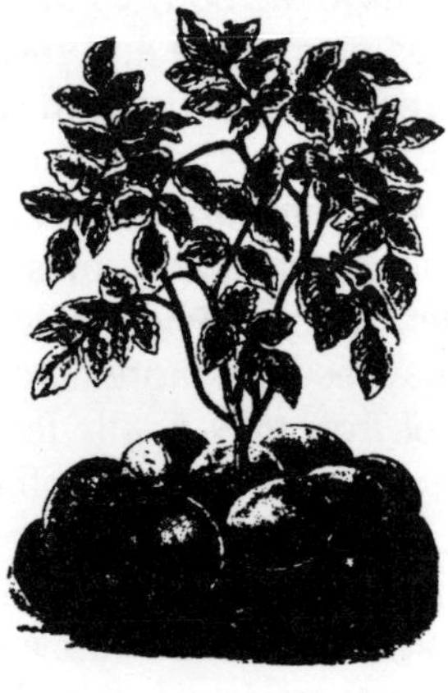

POTATO

How to Use Herbs

Remember, herbs cannot and do not cure by themselves, but they can and do hasten the process of elimination of toxic poisons that are the physical evidence of disease.

Diseases may be roughly classed as those under Common, Fixed, and Cardinal signs.

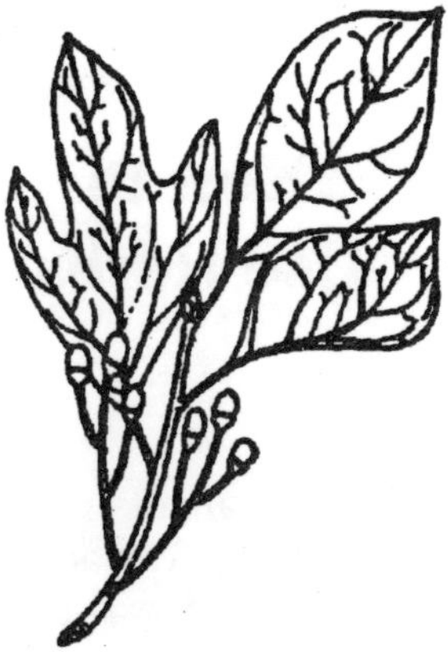

SASSAFRAS

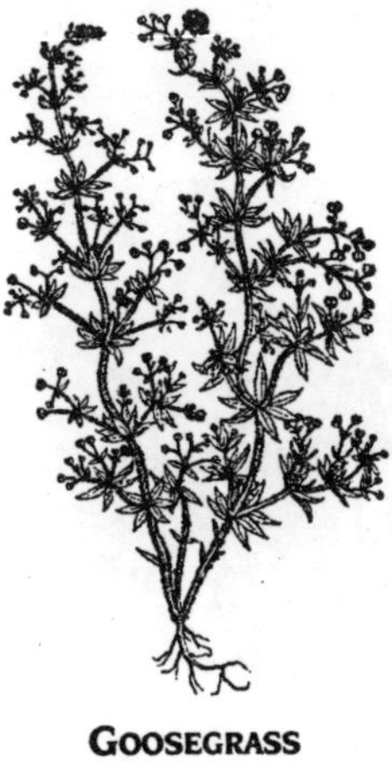

GOOSEGRASS

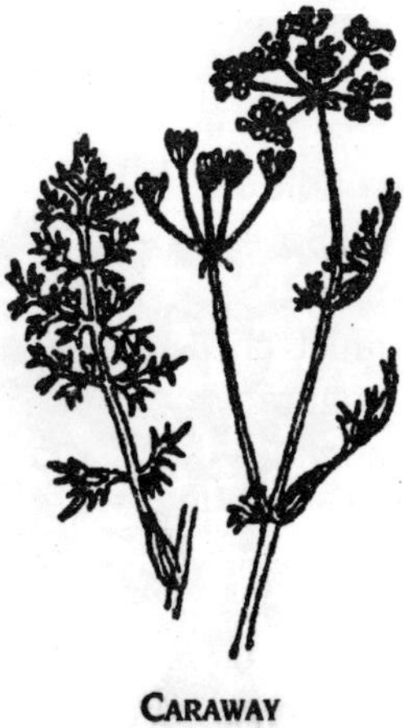

CARAWAY

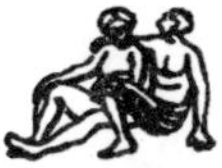
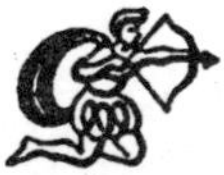

Herbs and Diseases of Common Signs

Under the Common signs, Gemini, Virgo, Sagittarius and Pisces, we have diseases of the respiratory organs which lead to liver and intestinal inactivity and nervous disorders.

To give a cough medicine may relieve the cough if it is sufficiently sedative, but to complete the cure, it must contain a liver tonic and a laxative.

To give a nervine may relieve neuritis and neuralgia for the time being, but we must also give something which will neutralize the acid condition of the blood.

So if we are seeking a remedy for any complaints coming under the Common signs we must choose from the herbs of Gemini, Virgo, Sagittarius, and Pisces those that will combine nervines, tonics, demulcents, and laxatives but either of these given alone may cause more harm than good.

The herbs under Gemini and Virgo which are most common are skullcap, valerian, celery, hops, cleavers, goosegrass, caraway, and endive. These are all nervines.

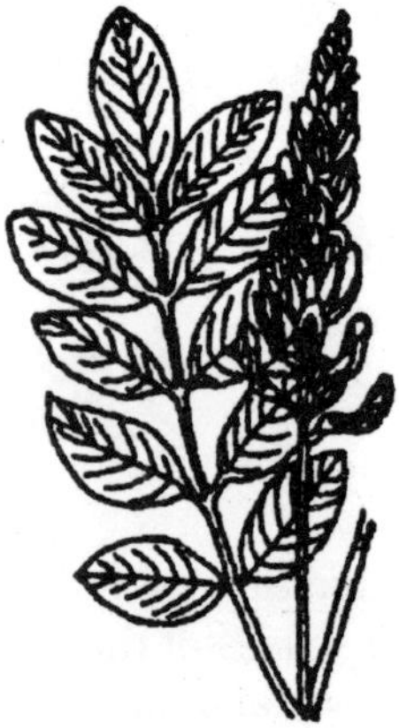

Licorice

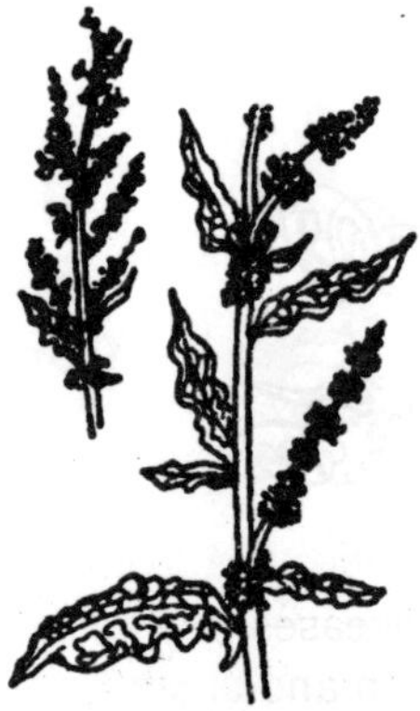

Yellowdock

The most common herbs under Sagittarius are red clover, sassafras, southernwood, bayberry, burdock, yellowdock, sage, horseradish, and dandelion. These have a tonic action on the liver and glandular system generally.

The herbs under Pisces are demulcent and the most common are: Iceland moss, consumption moss, coltsfoot, and skunk cabbage.

The laxatives, since they act upon the liver to increase and set free the bile, are also under Sagittarius and the best of these are Oregon grape and cascara bark. Licorice is a Mercurial laxative and is also nervine in its effect.

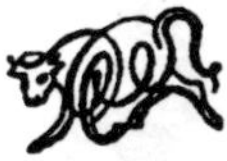
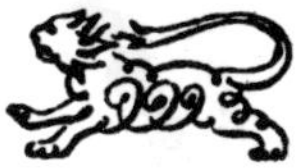

Herbs and Diseases of Fixed Signs

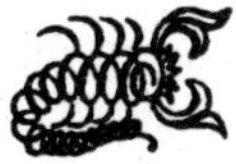
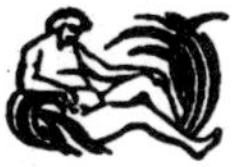

Diseases of the Fixed signs affect arterial circulation and are mainly the result of emotional disturbances. The lower brain and throat are under the rulership of Taurus, the heart under Leo, the generative organs under Scorpio, and the glands of the knees and ankles under Aquarius.

The herbs under Leo gently simulate the circulation; under Taurus they free the blood from excess water; under Scorpio they cleanse the blood of impurities; and under Aquarius the moisture in the body is controlled.

So complaints under the fixed signs call for stimulants to increase the circulation, sudorifics to keep the pores of the skin active, laxatives for intestinal activity, and sedatives to allay nervous excitement.

Under the rulership of Leo we have celandine, coltsfoot, chamomile, eyebright, juniper, marigold, pimpernel, rue, St. John's wort, walnut, and peppers.

Under Taurus we have apples, elder, dogdaisy, tansy, yarrow, marshmallow, ground ivy, plantain, and moss.

Under Scorpio we have horehound, broom, leeks, onions, rhubarb, nettles, butterbur, and under Aquarius the chief herbs are valerian and snakeroot.

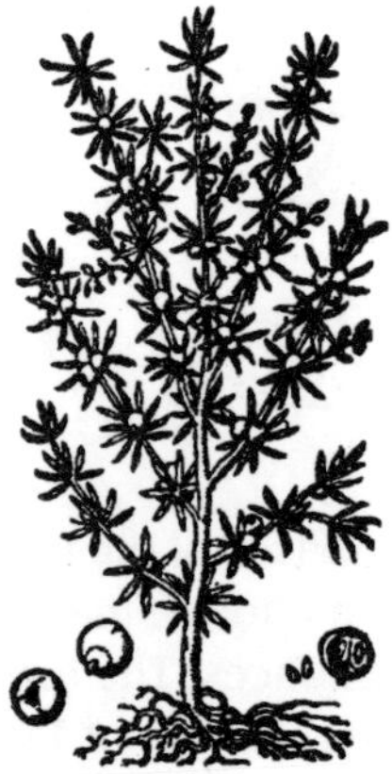

JUNIPER

It is best to combine the herbs of each of the above signs for complaints of the circulatory system. A tea made of broom may relieve Jaundice which is a Scorpio complaint, but it is better to add a little cayenne pepper as a stimulant, valerian as a nervine, and marshmallow as a demulcent.

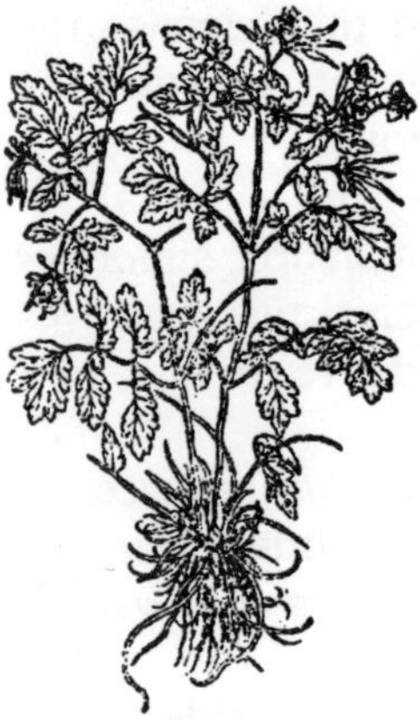

CELADINE

Asthma, a Leo complaint, may be relieved by coltsfoot, but if we add ground ivy, the pores of the skin are kept gently open and nettles will stimulate the circulation while snake root is a mild expectorant.

Cramp, an Aquarian affliction, may be relieved by cramp bark alone (a Scorpio herb), but juniper, yarrow, and valerian in small quantities also will increase its effectiveness.

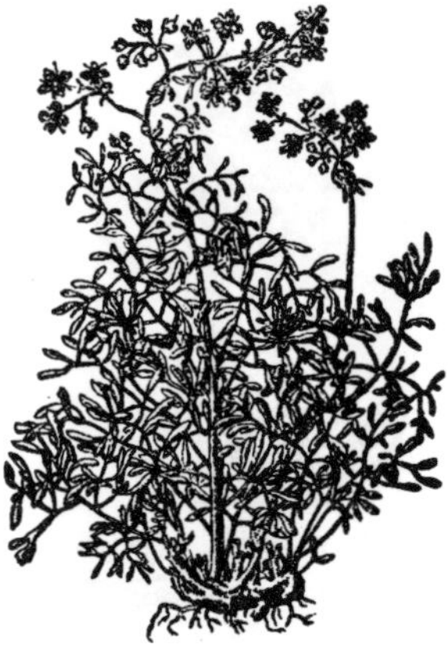

Rue

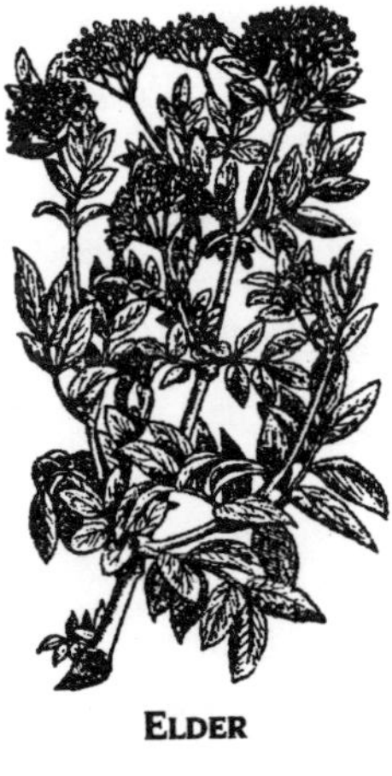

Elder

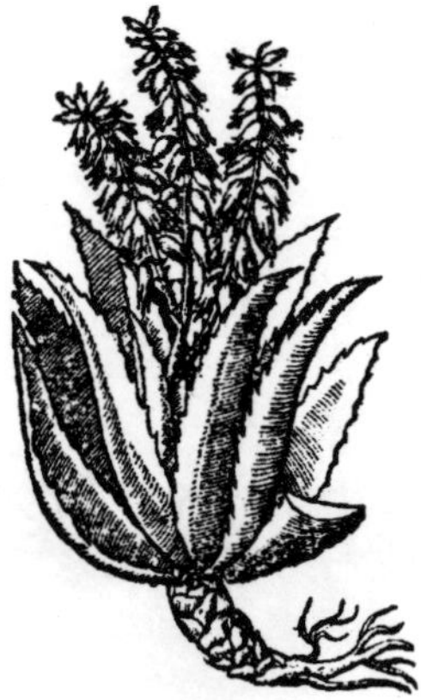

ALOE

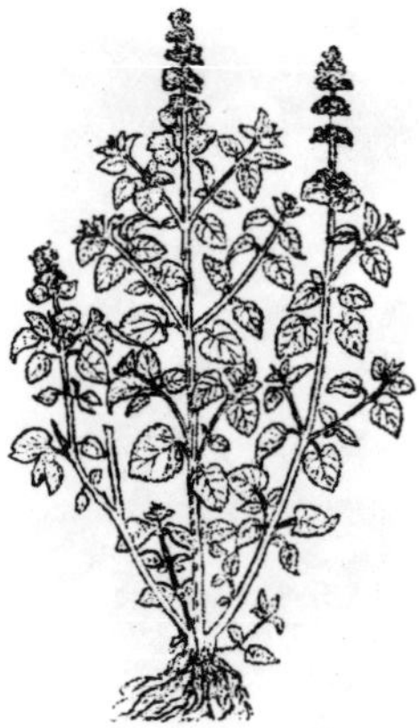

CATMINT

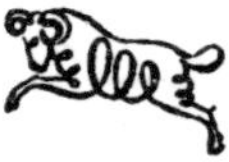

Herbs and Diseases of Cardinal Signs

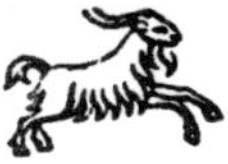

The diseases of the Cardinal signs are related to the venous circulation. The Cardinal signs, Aries, Cancer, Capricorn, and Libra tell of desires and ambitions connected with business, reputation, and home. An inharmony in any of these departments tends to produce disease in the head (Aries), stomach (Cancer), kidneys (Libra), and in the bones and skin (Capricorn).

The herbs then must be nervine for the head, stimulating for the stomach, harmonizing for the kidneys, and mucilaginous and astringent for the scrofulous skin.

The Aries herbs will be biting in taste and nervine, the commonest of these are allheal, aloes, catmint, gentian, garlic, ginger, land cress, mustard. The herbs of Cancer are chickweed, pumpkin seeds, lettuce, water cress, water violet. The herbs of Libra are balm, thyme, strawberry, violet. The herbs of Capricorn are comfrey, knotgrass, yellow cedar, and shepherd's purse.

In compounding herbs for complaints relating to the Cardinal signs, we must choose a Libra herb to neutralize the over-acidity, a Capricorn herb to give tone to the kidneys that the poisonous acids may be eliminated, a Cancer herb as a tonic to the stomach, and an Aries herb to soothe the nerves.

Herbs may be used fresh or dried and may be eaten in that condition. Barks are best if used when they are one year old and these are more powerful and bring results more quickly if they are chewed.

If cooked, the herbs should be made into a drink like ordinary tea and the barks and roots must be boiled for at least one hour, but it must be remembered that cooking tends to alter the nature of the herbs.

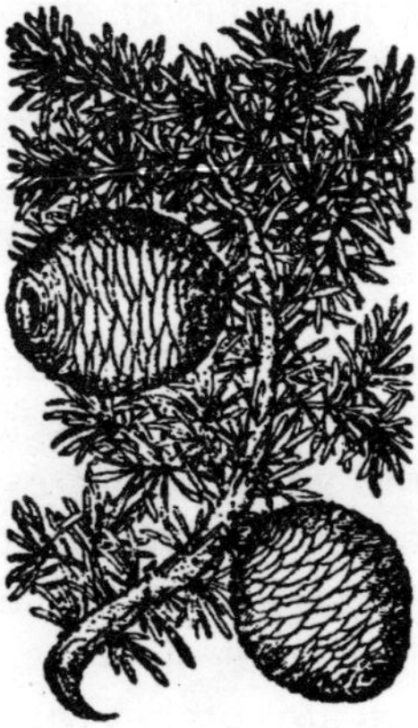

CEDAR

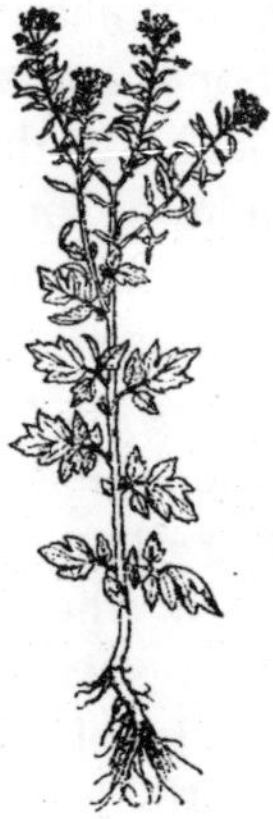

MUSTARD

BOOKS OF RELATED INTEREST

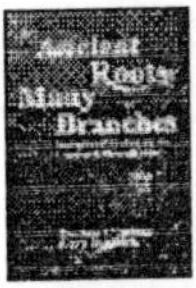

ANCIENT ROOTS, MANY BRANCHES
Energetics of Healing Across Cultures & Through Time
Darlena L'Orange & Gary Dolowich
ISBN: 978-81-7822-126-7

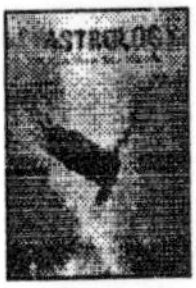

ASTROLOGY
A New Age Guide
Ed Perrone
ISBN: 978-81-7822-092-x

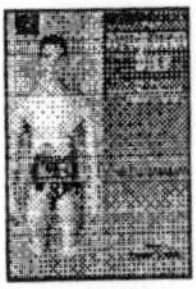

THE AYURVEDIC DIET
The Ancient Way to Health Rejuvenation and Weight Control
Dennis Thompson
ISBN: 978-81-7822-014-7

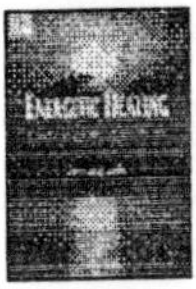

ENERGETIC HEALING
Embracing the Life Force
Arnie Lade
ISBN: 978-81-7822-005-5

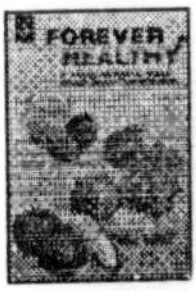

FOREVER HEALTHY
Preventing and Treating Disease through Timeless Natural Medicine
Kumuda Reddy & Stan Kendz
ISBN: 978-81-7822-171-7

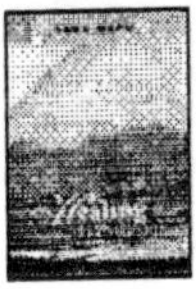

HEALING HANDBOOK
A spiritual guide to healing yourself and others
Tara Ward
ISBN: 978-81-7822-034-5

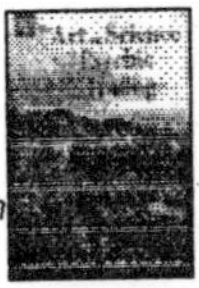

ART AND SCIENCE OF PSYCHIC HEALING
Larry & Phyllis G. McDaniel
ISBN: 978-81-7822-030-7

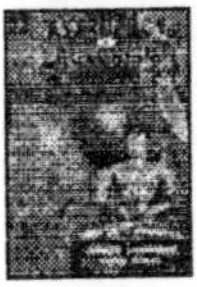

ASTROLOGY IN BUDDHISM
Buddhist Practice to Modern Astrology
Jhampa Shaneman & Jan V. Angel
ISBN: 978-81-7822-194-6

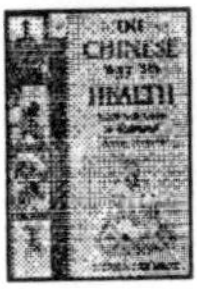

THE CHINESE WAY TO HEALTH
A Self-help guide to Traditional Chinese Medicine
Stephen Gascoigne
ISBN: 978-81-7822-160-1

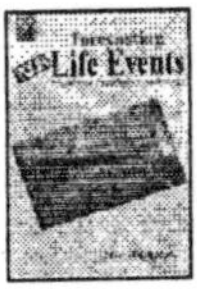

FORECASTING YOUR LIFE EVENTS
An Art of Predictive Astrology
Carol Rushman
ISBN: 978-81-7822-109-0

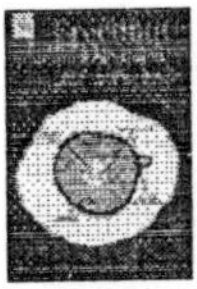

FREEDOM FROM DISEASE
How to Control Free Radicals, a Major Cause of Aging and Disease
Hari Sharma
ISBN: 978-81-7822-224-0

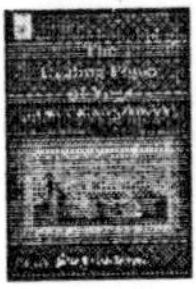

THE HEALING POWER OF YOGA
For Health, Well-Being and Inner Peace
Julie Friedeberger
ISBN: 978-81-7822-181-6

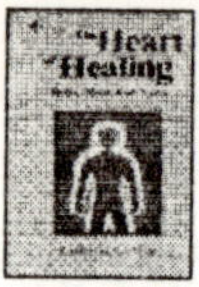

THE HEART OF HEALING
Body, Mind and Spirit

Caroline Latham

ISBN: 978-81-7822-019-2

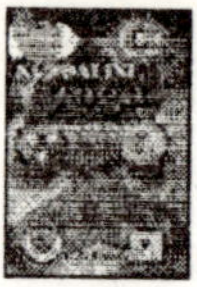

KUNDALINI YOGA
A Brief Study of Sir John Woodroff's "The Serpent Power"

M.P. Pandit

ISBN: 978-81-7822-076-5

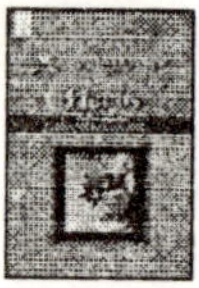

THE MAGICAL POWER OF HERBS
An Encyclopedia (Over 400 herbs described)
Scott Cunningham
ISBN: 978-81-7822-277-6

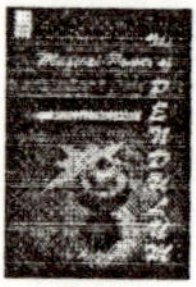

THE MAGICAL POWER OF PENDULUM
Focusing Your Energy for Self-Improvement & Psychic Development
Richard Webstar
ISBN: 978-81-7822-254-7

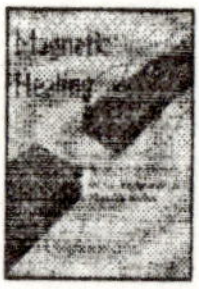

MAGNETIC HEALING
Advance Techniques for the Application of Magnetic Forces

Buryl Payne

ISBN: 978-81-7822-004-2

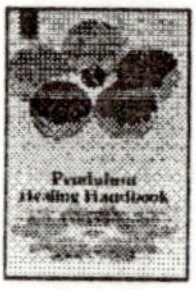

PENDULUM HEALING HANDBOOK

Walter Lübeck

ISBN: 978-81-7822-003-1

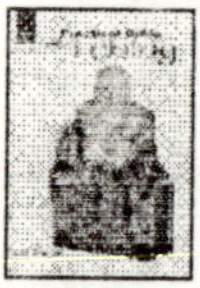

PRACTICAL GUIDE TO THE I CHING

Kim-Anh Lim

ISBN: 978-81-7822-108-3

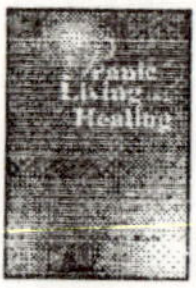

PRANIC LIVING AND HEALING

Luis S.R. Vas

ISBN: 978-81-7822-161-8

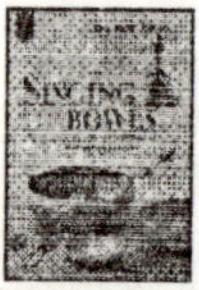

SINGING BOWLS
A Practical Handbook of Instruction and Use

Eva Rudy Jansen

ISBN: 978-81-7822-103-8

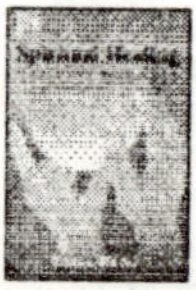

SPIRITUAL HEALING
Doctors Examine Therapeutic Touch and Other Holistic Treatments

Dora Kunz

ISBN: 978-81-7822-011-6

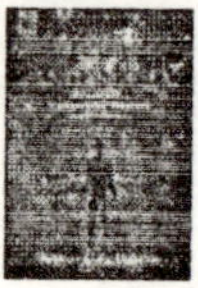

VEDIC ASTROLOGY
A Guide to the Fundamentals of Jyotish

Ronnie Gale Dreyer

ISBN: 978-81-7822-208-0

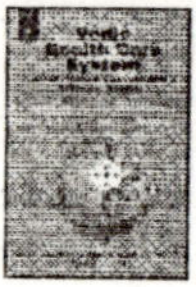

VEDIC HEALTH CARE SYSTEM
Clinical Practice of Sushrutokta Marm Chikitsa and Siravedhan

Ram Lal Sah, Binod & Geeta Joshi

ISBN: 978-81-7822-041-3